Praise for
Skinny **Bitch**

"A funny, foul-mouthed ode to adopting a vegan diet."
—Dwight Garner, *New York Times Book Review*

"The authors are brazen . . . They're not trying to win
popularity contests . . . they just want healthy people."
—Associated Press News Syndicate

"Ready to jump-start [the year] with an electric prod to the system? . . .
They tell it like it is, and without delicacy."
—*Chicago Sun Times*

"There's more solid advice in *Skinny Bitch* than in most diet and health books."
—*Bitch Magazine*

"By no means for the faint hearted . . . this is as hard hitting as it comes!"
—*Hot Stars* (UK)

"This diet book doesn't sugar-coat what you have to do to lose weight."
—*Grazia*

"It made me laugh . . ." —*Marie Claire UK*

"Sensible advice . . ." —*Health & Fitness UK*

" . . . an absolutely hilarious read . . . refreshingly in-your-face funny. . . .
What are you waiting for, you moron? Go buy this book!"
—*Florida Today*

"What makes this diet easy to swallow is the book's tough-love attitude—
part best-friend counsel, part drill-sergeant abuse and a dash of
sailor mouth, wrapped in a pretty chick-lit package."
—iVillage, Diet & Fitness

Skinny
Bitch
In the Kitch

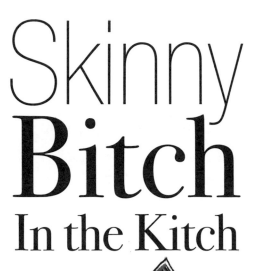

*Kick-ass recipes for
hungry girls who want
to stop cooking crap
(and start looking hot!)*

by Rory Freedman and Kim Barnouin

RUNNING PRESS
PHILADELPHIA · LONDON

9 8 7 6 5 4 3 2 1
Digit on the right indicates the number of this printing

Library of Congress Control Number: 2007933176

ISBN: 978-0-7624-3542-5

Book design by Amanda Richmond
Edited by Jennifer Kasius
Typography: Bodoni and Helvetica Neue

This book may be ordered by mail from the publisher.
Please include $2.50 for postage and handling.
But try your bookstore first!

Running Press Book Publishers
2300 Chestnut Street
Philadelphia, PA 19103-4371

Visit us on the web!
www.runningpress.com

To the truth-speakers and seekers who paved the way for us,
For the health food pioneers who blazed a trail for us to follow,
For our fellow foodies who love to eat as much as we do,
And for all the newly hatched Skinny Bitches who asked for this book.

Namastè.

CONTENTS

ACKNOWLEDGMENTS

Jill Hough, we cannot imagine what this book would be without your passion, dedication, and culinary brilliance. Thank you! Talia Cohen, Jennifer Kasius, Amanda Richmond, Seta Bedrossian Zink, Craig Herman, and Victoria Gilder: For your ceaseless support and enthusiasm and for everything you do (including the things you do that we'll never even know about), we express our sincerest gratitude. Really. We are so thankful for each of you. For creating the perfect *Skinny Bitch*, we will forever be indebted to you, Margarete Gockel. Chloe Jo Berman, Talia Berman, Karen Coyne, Meri Freedman, Bruce Friedrich, Jessica Jonas, Dave and Linda Middlesworth, Jack Norris, Steve Perron, Gretchen Ryan, Lauren and Tracy Silverman, and everyone at VTM: Your commitment and generosity leave us in awe. And to everyone at Laura Dail Literary Agency, Perseus Books, and Running Press: We humbly thank each of you for being part of the collective that makes this all possible. We don't take any of you for granted.

For our friends and families, who make the whole journey a joy— we couldn't ask for more.

INTRODUCTION

What's better than eating? (If you say "sex," you're either a liar or a pervert.) The answer is: Nothing! There's nothing better than eating! We're total pigs and eating is, without a doubt, our favorite thing to do. We love eating so much, it makes us mad. We have, like, a violent passion for food. When we go out to eat, if something we order is really good, we talk about killing the chef. Or our pets. Or ourselves. Good food makes us want to die . . . you know, like that expression, ". . . to die for." But ironically, we also care about our health.

It was these two things—our obsessive passion for food and our concern for health—that led us to write *Skinny Bitch*. If you haven't read *Skinny Bitch* yet, get your head out of your ass and go buy a copy. It will change your life. Seriously. Don't be fooled by the title; it's not some dumb, fluffy, weight-loss book. It's a comprehensive guide on how to eat well *and* enjoy food. But it's also a well-researched exposé documenting the shady business surrounding what we eat.

Much of what we learned while researching *Skinny Bitch* blew our minds. So we've made it our personal mission to share this information. We wanted to reprint *Skinny Bitch* in its entirety right here in the introduction, but our whore publisher wouldn't let us. So we're gonna give you the Cliff Notes . . .

Meat:

Hmm . . . dead, rotting, decomposing flesh of carcasses. Doesn't sound like something you'd want to eat, huh? Not to mention the pesticides, hormones, steroids, and antibiotics. Oops! We almost forgot mad cow disease, bird flu, salmonella, E. coli, trichinosis, and mercury. Well, no wonder Americans are suffering from obesity; cancer; liver, kidney, lung, and reproductive disorders; birth defects; miscarriages; and nervous system disorders.

You can call it steak, tuna, bacon, or chicken. No matter how you slice it, it's a piece of decaying, decomposing carcass. We know you like the taste, but there are other foods out there that mimic the flavor and texture of meat but don't come with the same side effects. Smarten up, bitches.

Dairy:

Got osteoporosis? Researchers at Harvard, Yale, Penn State, and the National Institutes of Health have studied the effects of dairy intake on bones. Not one of these studies found dairy to be a deterrent to osteoporosis. On the contrary, a study funded by the National Dairy Council itself revealed that the high protein content of milk actually leaches calcium from the body. These findings are consistent with many others that blame milk not only for osteoporosis, but also acne, anemia, anxiety, ADD, allergies, asthma, obesity, heart disease, diabetes, autism, and multiple cancers.

Just like human milk is for baby humans, cows' milk is for baby cows. We're the only species on the planet that drinks the milk of another species. We're also the only species on the planet that drinks milk as adults. It's not only gross, it's creepy. We've been totally duped by the dairy industry and their hundreds of millions of advertising dollars. And now we're totally addicted to their disease-causing products.

There's no need for any of them. It's the new millennium. There are so many awesome alternatives to dairy products. Get with the program, bitches.

Carbs:

There is so much bullshit around carbs now; we've got to set the record straight. There are two types of carbs—simple and complex. Complex carbs are not only good for you, but they're a vital part of your diet. They consist of fruits, vegetables, whole grains, and legumes, and they should be eaten all day, every day. Simple carbs suck and should be avoided: white bread, white flour, white pasta, white rice, and white sugar. Most cookies, cakes, snacks, and processed foods are simple carbs.

So what's a pig to do? Have her cake and eat it—just make the cake with good ingredients. Duh!

Whenever we do interviews promoting *Skinny Bitch*, we're always asked the same questions: "What do you do when you get cravings for cookies? Or does that never happen to Skinny Bitches?" Um, we're Skinny Bitches, not aliens! Of course we get cravings for cookies. And when we do, we eat 'em!

Unfortunately, most people have no idea that they can truly enjoy food without getting fat, sick, or sad. So it's our pleasure (oink, oink) to educate and feed the masses. We hope you'll love these recipes as much as we do. If you don't, go have sex, you pervert.

Bitchclaimer

There's nothing more annoying than recipes with a million obscure ingredients. So we tried to make all our recipes as "normal" as possible. However, there are a few products we insist on using, despite their potential to peeve you. You may not have whole wheat flour lying around in your cupboard, but too bad. White flour is crap for your body and should only be used when absolutely necessary. Whenever we can, we use products that are as pure and healthy as possible. And we want the same for you. We want you to replace your old, shitty ingredients and start eating better.

Now granted, there's nothing wrong with olive oil. In fact, we love it. But did you know that when you heat most oils at high temperatures, you change their molecular structures, causing free-radicals? And that free-radicals have been linked to heart disease and cancer? Well, we knew that (we're really smart), so a lot of our recipes call for coconut oil instead. Yeah, you may have to go to a health food store to buy it, but isn't a trip to the health food store better than a trip to the Emergency Room?

So if you come across a few ingredients that irritate you: Don't hate. Appreciate. We love you and we want you to enjoy food *and* be healthy. We have a glossary in the back to explain some of the funky stuff. So quit your bitching, restock your cabinets, and get cookin'.

(Don't worry, though—there are some naughty, crappy ingredients in here, too.)

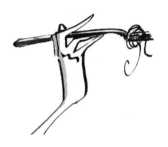

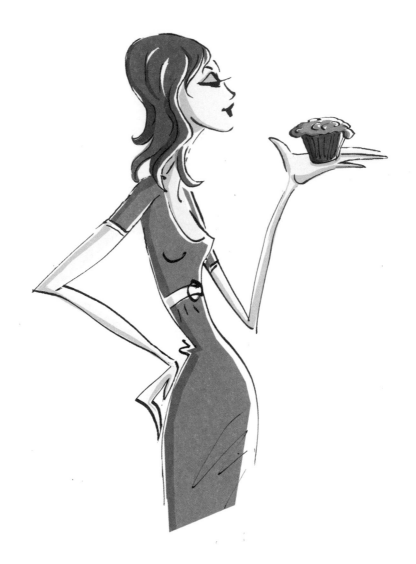

Bitchin'
BREAKFASTS

*Coffee sucks for your body and is no way to start
your day. (If that's news to you, go read* Skinny Bitch,
*pages 15–16.) The real breakfast of champions is
fresh fruit. But for weekend brunches and those days when
fruit ain't gonna cut it, enjoy these bitchin' breakfasts.*

French Scramble

Homemade Granola Parfait

THE Breakfast Sandwich

Potato Scramble

Pecan-crusted French Toast

Basic Pancakes

Basic Fruit and Nut Muffins

Smoothies

Bitchin' Breakfast Burrito

Denver Bitchlette for Two

French Scramble

Serves 3 or 4

14 to 16 ounces firm or extra firm tofu, crumbled (use your hands or a fork)

4 ounces vegan Jack, cheddar, or American cheese, shredded

3 scallions, sliced

2 cloves garlic, minced

2 tablespoons nutritional yeast flakes

1 tablespoon tamari or soy sauce

½ teaspoon turmeric

½ teaspoon fine sea salt

½ teaspoon pepper

½ tablespoon refined coconut oil

1 cup sliced mushrooms (any kind, or a combination)

2 cups fresh spinach leaves

In a large bowl, combine the tofu, cheese, scallions, garlic, yeast flakes, tamari or soy sauce, turmeric, salt, and pepper. Set aside.

In a large nonstick skillet over medium heat, melt the coconut oil. Add the mushrooms and cook, stirring occasionally, until tender, about 1½ minutes. Stir in the spinach, a handful at a time if necessary, and cook until wilted, about 1 minute. Stir in the tofu mixture and cook, stirring occasionally, for 3 to 4 minutes, or until any liquid has evaporated and the mixture is hot. Serve immediately.

Homemade Granola Parfait

Makes 1

1 cup berries (if using strawberries,
    hull and quarter them)

1 (6-ounce) container vanilla
    or fruit-flavored soy yogurt

⅔ cup homemade granola

HOMEMADE GRANOLA

Makes about 6 cups

2 cups rolled oats

1¼ cups (4 ounces) sliced almonds

¾ cup unsweetened
    shredded coconut

¼ teaspoon fine sea salt

¼ cup maple syrup

2 tablespoons rice syrup

2 tablespoons safflower oil, plus
    more for greasing baking sheet

1 cup dried fruit (raisins, golden
    raisins, cranberries, chopped
    apricots — use just one or any
    combination you want)

Preheat oven to 300°F.

Arrange the oats on a large rimmed baking sheet and bake, stirring occasionally, until lightly toasted, about 15 minutes.

Meanwhile, in a large bowl, combine the almonds, coconut, and salt. In a small bowl, whisk together the maple syrup, rice syrup, and oil.

Stir the toasted oats into the almond mixture. Add the syrup mixture, stirring to thoroughly combine.

Grease the baking sheet. Spread the granola evenly on the sheet and bake, stirring occasionally, until golden brown, 20 to 25 minutes (the mixture will still look and feel wet). Stir in the dried fruit, then cool completely in the pan on a wire rack. (It'll be torturous waiting for it to cool. But do your best. This bitch is hot.) Store in an airtight container.

THE Breakfast Sandwich

Makes 4

1 (7- or 8-ounce) package
baked or fried tofu (2 squares)
2 tablespoons refined coconut oil
4 slices vegan Canadian bacon
or ham
4 slices vegan Jack, cheddar,
or American cheese
4 whole wheat English muffins,
split and toasted
4 slices tomato (optional)
2 tablespoons soy butter
Fine sea salt
Pepper
Ketchup (optional)

Halve both of the tofu squares crosswise, making 4 patties. In a large skillet over medium heat, melt the coconut oil. Add the tofu and bacon or ham and cook 2 minutes. Turn both and add a small amount of soy butter to the tofu before topping the tofu with the cheese. Cover and cook another 2 minutes. On each of the 4 muffin bottoms, arrange 1 slice of bacon or ham, 1 piece of tofu with cheese, and 1 slice of tomato, if using. Sprinkle generously with salt and pepper, add ketchup if desired, and add the muffin tops. Serve immediately. Then die happy.

Potato Scramble

Serves 4 to 6

8 ounces vegan Jack, cheddar, or mozzarella cheese, shredded

7 to 8 ounces firm or extra firm tofu, cut into ½-inch dice

2 tomatoes, cut into ½-inch dice

1 teaspoon fine sea salt

½ teaspoon pepper

½ teaspoon paprika

1 tablespoon refined coconut oil

8 ounces vegan breakfast sausage, crumbled or cut into small bite-sized pieces

½ onion, cut into ½-inch dice

2 russet potatoes (about 24 ounces), cut into ½-inch dice

2 cloves garlic, thinly sliced

In a large bowl, combine the cheese, tofu, tomatoes, salt, pepper, and paprika; set aside.

In a large nonstick skillet over medium heat, melt ½ tablespoon of the coconut oil. Add the sausage and cook according to package directions. Transfer the sausage to the bowl with the cheese mixture. Add the remaining ½ tablespoon of coconut oil to the skillet and melt over medium heat. Add the onion and cook, stirring occasionally, for 1 minute. Add the potatoes and cook, stirring occasionally, until the potato is tender, 15 to 20 minutes. Stir in the garlic and cook for 1 minute. Stir in the cheese mixture and cook, stirring occasionally, for 2 to 3 minutes, or until the mixture is hot.

Pecan-crusted French Toast

Makes 6 to 8 slices

1½ cups soy or rice milk

3 tablespoons corn starch

1 teaspoon cinnamon

6 tablespoons chickpea flour
or brown rice flour

1 cup finely chopped pecans

2 tablespoons refined coconut oil,
or more as needed for cooking

6 to 8 slices vegan whole wheat
or whole wheat raisin bread

Maple syrup, for serving

In a medium bowl, whisk together the soy or rice milk, corn starch, and cinnamon. Whisk in the chickpea or brown rice flour. Transfer the mixture to a shallow bowl. Place the pecans in another shallow bowl.

In a large skillet over medium heat, melt the coconut oil. One slice at a time, dip the bread in the milk mixture, turning to soak both sides. Dip one side in the pecans, pressing to coat. (Yeah, it's a little challenging to make 'em stick in there. Quit whining. You're about to have French toast!) Arrange the bread in the skillet (you might have to do more than one batch), pecan side down. Cook 2 to 3 minutes, until the pecans are well browned. Carefully turn the bread and continue cooking until the second side is browned, 2 to 3 minutes. Serve immediately with maple syrup.

Basic Pancakes

**Makes about eight
4- to 5-inch pancakes**

1¼ cups whole wheat pastry flour

1½ teaspoons baking powder

½ teaspoon fine sea salt

1½ cups rice milk

2 tablespoons refined coconut oil,
    melted, or safflower oil

1 tablespoon maple syrup,
    plus more for serving

1 teaspoon pure vanilla extract

In a large bowl, whisk together the flour, baking powder, and salt. In a medium bowl, whisk together the rice milk, oil, maple syrup, and vanilla. Whisk the milk mixture into the flour mixture, stirring just until combined (a few lumps are okay).

Preheat a nonstick griddle or large nonstick skillet over medium heat for at least 2 minutes. About ¼ cup at a time, pour the batter onto the grill or skillet. Cook until bubbles appear, the edges are set, and the pancakes are nicely browned on the bottom (about 2 to 3 minutes). Turn and cook until the other side is nicely browned, 1 to 2 minutes. If necessary, keep the finished pancakes in a warm oven while you finish the batter. Serve hot with maple syrup.

BLUEBERRY PANCAKES
Stir 1 cup of blueberries into the batter.

BANANA WALNUT PANCAKES
Stir 1 large banana, thinly sliced, and ½ cup chopped walnuts into the batter.

CHOCOLATE PANCAKES
Reduce the whole-wheat pastry flour to 1 cup plus 2 tablespoons. Add ¼ cup unsweetened cocoa powder. Increase the syrup to 2 tablespoons.

Basic Fruit and Nut Muffins

Makes 12 standard-sized muffins

¼ cup refined coconut oil, melted, or safflower oil, plus more for greasing muffin tins

2 cups whole wheat pastry flour

½ cup Sucanat or other dry sweetener

1 tablespoon Ener-G egg replacer

2 teaspoons baking powder

¼ teaspoon fine sea salt

1¼ cups soy milk

1 teaspoon vanilla

1 cup fresh or dried fruit, diced or chunked, if necessary

½ cup chopped nuts (optional)

Preheat oven to 375°F. Grease a standard-sized muffin tin or use muffin liners.

In a large bowl, combine the pastry flour, Sucanat, baking powder, salt and egg replacer. In a medium bowl, whisk together the soy milk, oil, and vanilla. Add the milk mixture to the flour mixture, stirring until barely combined. Stir in the fruit and nuts, if using. Transfer the batter to the prepared muffin tin, dividing it evenly. Bake for 15 to 20 minutes, or until a toothpick inserted into the center of the muffins comes out clean.

CRANBERRY ORANGE MUFFINS

Add the zest of ½ orange. Use dried cranberries for the fruit and omit the nuts.

TROPICAL MACADAMIA NUT MUFFINS

Add the zest of ½ orange, combine banana and shredded coconut for the fruit, and use macadamias for the nuts.

APPLE CINNAMON MUFFINS

Use apples for the fruit, omit the nuts, and add 1 teaspoon ground cinnamon, ¼ teaspoon ground nutmeg, and ⅛ teaspoon ground cloves to the dry ingredients.

ZUCCHINI RAISIN MUFFINS

Combine shredded zucchini and raisins for the fruit, omit the nuts, and add 1 teaspoon ground cinnamon and ½ teaspoon ground ginger to the dry ingredients.

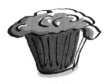

Basic Fruit Smoothie

Makes about 2 cups

2 cups chunked, frozen fruit
(see note)

1 cup soy milk or juice OR ½ cup
soy milk and ½ cup juice

In a blender, combine the fruit and soy milk and/or juice. Puree until smooth.

> If using fresh fruit, just add ½ cup ice cubes.

STRAWBERRY BANANA SMOOTHIE

Use a banana and strawberries for the fruit, and all soy milk for the liquid.

VERY BERRY SMOOTHIE

Use mixed berries for the fruit, and half soy milk, half apple juice for the liquid. (Or you can use all soy milk.)

JUST PEACHY SMOOTHIE

Use peaches for the fruit, and half soy milk, half apple juice for the liquid.

TROPICAL ORANGE GINGER SMOOTHIE

Use banana for the fruit, and orange juice for the liquid; add 1 tablespoon minced fresh ginger.

Bitchin' Breakfast Burrito

Makes 4

14 to 16 ounces firm or extra firm tofu,
  crumbled (use your hands or a fork)

2 cloves garlic, minced

2 tablespoons nutritional yeast flakes

1 tablespoon tamari or soy sauce

½ teaspoon turmeric

1 teaspoon fine sea salt

½ teaspoon pepper

1 tablespoon refined coconut oil

8 ounces vegan breakfast sausage,
  crumbled

1 russet potato (about 12 ounces),
  cut into ½-inch dice

1 (15-ounce) can black or pinto
  beans, drained

1 (4-ounce) can diced green chiles,
  drained

4 (9- to 10-inch) whole wheat tortillas,
  heated

4 ounces vegan cheddar or Jack
  cheese, shredded

1½ to 2 cups salsa

In a large bowl, combine the tofu, garlic, yeast flakes, tamari or soy sauce, turmeric, salt, and pepper; set aside.

In a large nonstick skillet over medium heat, melt ½ tablespoon of the coconut oil. Add the sausage and cook according to package directions. Transfer the sausage to the bowl with the tofu mixture. Add the remaining ½ tablespoon of coconut oil to the skillet and melt over medium heat. Add the potato and cook, stirring occasionally, until tender, 12 to 15 minutes. Add the beans and chiles, stirring until heated through, about 1 minute. Stir in the tofu mixture and cook, stirring occasionally, for 3 to 4 minutes, or until any liquid has evaporated and the mixture is hot.

To serve, lay a tortilla on a work surface and top with ¼ of the tofu mixture, arranging it in a column down the middle of the tortilla, 2 inches from either edge. Top with ¼ of the cheese and ¼ cup of the salsa. Fold one side of the tortilla up and over the fillings, fold in the edges, and continue rolling the tortilla to the other side, making a tight bundle. Transfer the burrito to a plate, seam down. Repeat with remaining tortillas. Pass the remaining salsa at the table. Olé, bitches!

Denver Bitchlette for Two

Serves 2

9 to 10 ounces firm or extra firm tofu, crumbled (use your hands or a fork)

3 ounces vegan Jack, cheddar, or American cheese, shredded

2 cloves garlic, minced

4 teaspoons nutritional yeast flakes

2 teaspoons tamari or soy sauce

2 teaspoons Ener-G egg replacer

½ teaspoon turmeric

½ teaspoon fine sea salt

½ teaspoon pepper

1 tablespoon refined coconut oil

½ green bell pepper, cut into ¼-inch dice

½ red bell pepper, cut into ¼-inch dice

¼ onion, cut into ¼-inch dice

1 slice or about 1 ounce vegan Canadian bacon or ham, cut into ¼-inch dice

Paprika for garnish (optional)

In a large bowl, combine the tofu, cheese, garlic, yeast flakes, tamari or soy sauce, egg replacer, turmeric, salt, and pepper. Set aside.

In a large nonstick skillet over medium heat, melt ½ tablespoon of the coconut oil. Add the green bell pepper, red bell pepper, and onion and cook, stirring occasionally, until tender, about 3 minutes. Transfer the vegetables to a plate or bowl.

Return the skillet to medium heat and melt the remaining ½ tablespoon of coconut oil. Add the tofu mixture and cook, stirring occasionally, for 2 minutes. Then spread it evenly in the pan and cook, without stirring, until nicely browned on the bottom, 2 to 3 minutes.

Arrange the vegetable mixture and bacon or ham on top of one side of the omelet. Remove from the heat and gently slide the omelet about halfway onto a serving plate. Carefully turn the pan over to fold the omelet in half on the plate.

Don't get all cranky if you screw up folding the Bitch-lette. It's definitely a talent that takes time to develop.

If you want, sprinkle the omelet with paprika before serving.

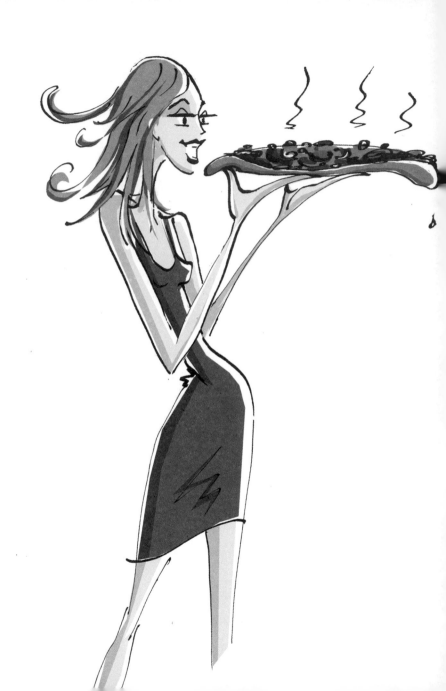

PMS
PISSY MOOD
SNACKS

If a group of scientists conducted a study
saying PMS wasn't "real," we'd kill them all.
Then we'd stuff our faces like sows.
This is what we'd eat.

Quesadillas

"Ham" and Cheese Puff Pockets

Onion Rings

Oven-Baked Garlic Fries

Quick Tortilla Pizzas

Quesadillas with Beans, Soy Cheese, Guacamole, and Salsa

Serves 2 as an entree

or 4 as an appetizer

½ tablespoon refined coconut oil
(optional)

2 (9- or 10-inch) whole wheat
flour tortillas

5 ounces vegan Jack or cheddar
cheese (or a combination), shredded

⅓ cup drained black or pinto beans

½ cup prepared salsa

¼ cup guacamole, homemade
or store bought (recipe follows)

Spread the coconut oil, if using, on one side of each tortilla, dividing it evenly. Lay the tortillas, oiled side down if applicable, on a work surface. Arrange the cheese on top, dividing it evenly, covering only half of the tortilla and leaving a 1-inch border at the edge. Arrange the beans and 2 tablespoons of the salsa on top of the cheese, dividing them evenly. Fold the tortillas in half.

In a large nonstick skillet over medium heat, cook the quesadillas, covered, until golden brown, about 4 minutes. Flip the quesadillas and cook, uncovered, until the second side is golden brown and the cheese has melted, about 2 minutes. Cut the quesadillas in wedges and transfer to serving plates or a platter. Top with guacamole and a spoonful of the remaining salsa. Pass any leftover salsa at the table.

GUACAMOLE

Makes about 1 cup

1 medium avocado

1 clove garlic, minced or pressed

Juice of ½ lime (about 1 tablespoon)

½ teaspoon fine sea salt

In a small bowl, use a potato masher or fork to combine the avocado, garlic, lime, and salt, stirring to make a coarse purée. Use immediately.

"Ham" and Cheese Puff Pockets

Makes 4

Whole wheat pastry flour,
    for dusting work surface

2 (9-inch) vegan whole wheat pie
    crusts, room temperature

4 ounces vegan cheddar cheese,
    shredded

4 ounces vegan sliced ham

Preheat oven to 400°F. Line a rimmed baking sheet with parchment.

On a work surface lightly dusted with whole wheat pastry flour, combine both pie crusts and roll them into a 12 x 12-inch rectangle. Cut the pastry in quarters to make four 6-inch squares. Top the squares with about half of the cheese, dividing evenly, covering only half of the pastry and leaving a ¾-inch border at the edge. Fold or cut the ham to cover the cheese, dividing evenly. Place the remaining cheese on top of the ham, dividing evenly.

Fold the pastry in half, pressing the edges together to seal in the filling. Crimp the edges with a fork. Prick the pocket a few times to create air vents. Transfer the pockets to the prepared baking sheet and bake for 20 minutes or until nicely browned.

Onion Rings

Makes about 20 rings

Refined coconut oil,
   for greasing baking sheet
1 onion (preferably a sweet
   type), cut crosswise into
   ⅓-inch-thick slices
½ cup seasoned whole
   wheat bread crumbs
½ cup cornmeal
1 teaspoon fine sea salt,
   plus more for sprinkling
¾ cup rice flour
¾ cup soy or rice milk
Ketchup, or other dipping
   sauce (optional)

Preheat oven to 450°F. Grease a large rimmed baking sheet; set aside.

Separate the onion slices into rings and pick out 20 or so of the largest (reserve the rest for another use). In a shallow bowl, combine the bread crumbs, cornmeal, and salt. Place the rice flour in a second bowl and the soy milk in a third. One at a time, dip the onion rings in the soy milk, the rice flour, the soy milk again, and then the bread crumb mixture, pressing to thoroughly coat. Arrange the coated rings on the prepared baking sheet and bake for 25 to 30 minutes, or until nicely browned. Sprinkle with salt and serve with ketchup, if desired.

Oven-baked Garlic Fries

Serves 3 or 4

2 russet potatoes, scrubbed,
   peeled (if desired), and cut
   into ¼-inch sticks

4½ tablespoons refined coconut
   oil, melted, or safflower oil

4 cloves garlic, minced

Fine sea salt

1 teaspoon chopped fresh
   parsley (optional)

> * Don't be cheap with the
> baking sheets, even though
> you might be able to squeeze
> them onto just one. More
> room around the fries helps
> them crisp.

Preheat oven to 450°F.

In a large bowl, combine the potatoes with 3 tablespoons of the oil, tossing to coat evenly. Arrange the potatoes on two* large rimmed baking sheets in a single layer and bake for 15 minutes. One pan at a time, remove the fries from the oven and flip them over with a spatula. Rearrange the fries in a single layer and return them to the oven for 15 to 20 minutes, until crisp outside and cooked through.

Meanwhile, in a small saucepan over low heat, combine the remaining 1½ tablespoons of oil and the garlic. Cook, stirring occasionally, until the garlic is fragrant and starting to brown, about 3 minutes.

Transfer the fries to serving plates or a platter. Sprinkle generously with salt and drizzle with the garlic mixture. Sprinkle with parsley, if desired.

Quick Tortilla Pizzas

Makes 4

4 (9- to 10-inch) whole wheat tortillas

1 cup Roasted Red Pepper Sauce
(recipe below)

4 to 6 ounces vegan mozzarella,
shredded

½ small red onion, thinly sliced

⅓ cup halved and pitted
Kalamata olives

2 cups loosely packed arugula,
(optional)

Preheat oven to 475°F.

Arrange tortillas on two rimmed baking sheets. *

Top the tortillas with the Roasted Red Pepper Sauce, cheese, onion, and olives, dividing evenly. Bake for 8 to 10 minutes, until the cheese is bubbly and the edges are brown.

Cut the pizzas into quarters, top with the arugula, if using, and serve.

ROASTED RED PEPPER SAUCE

Makes 1 cup

1 cup drained jarred roasted
red peppers

6 large basil leaves

¼ teaspoon fine sea salt

⅛ teaspoon pepper

In the bowl of a food processor, combine the roasted red peppers, basil, tomato paste, salt, and pepper; pulse to form a coarse paste.

* For crispy pizza, bake the tortillas for 3 minutes, flip 'em and bake 'em for 3 minutes more. Then, add the toppings and bake for 8 to 10 minutes.

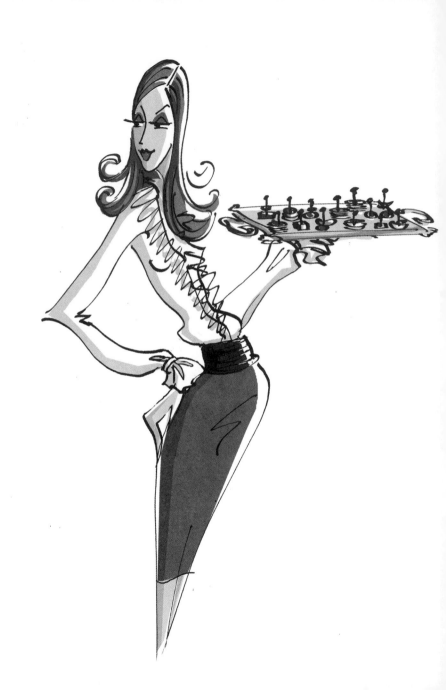

Grown-up
APPETIZERS

*If we were having a dinner party
and pretending to be classy,
we'd make stuff like this.*

Crabby Cakes with Remoulade Sauce

Garlicky White Bean Spread on Crostini

Herbed "Egg" Salad Scoops

Mock Chopped Liver

Spicy Mixed Nuts

Stuffed Mushrooms

Spicy Sushi Rolls
with Avocado and Cucumber

Crabby Cakes with Remoulade Sauce

Serves 8 as an appetizer

(or 4 as an entrée)

About 2 tablespoons refined
   coconut oil

1 cup diced carrots

½ cup diced celery

4 shallots, minced

2 cups finely shredded parsnip

1 cup whole wheat panko
   (Japanese-style bread crumbs)
   or whole wheat bread crumbs

¼ cup chickpea flour
   or brown rice flour

2 tablespoons Ener-G egg replacer

4 teaspoons kelp powder

1½ teaspoons fine sea salt

¼ teaspoon pepper

½ cup vegan mayonnaise

About 1 cup Remoulade Sauce
   (recipe follows)

In a large nonstick skillet, heat 1 tablespoon of the coconut oil. Add the carrots and celery and cook over medium heat, stirring occasionally, for 2 minutes. Add the shallots and cook, stirring occasionally, for 1 minute, or until all the vegetables are tender. Remove from heat and allow to cool.

In a mixing bowl, combine the parsnip, panko, flour, egg replacer, kelp powder, salt, and pepper. Stir in the carrot and celery mixture and mayonnaise. Shape the mixture into 8 cakes, about 3 inches across and ¾ inch thick.

Wipe out the skillet and return it to medium heat. Add the remaining tablespoon of coconut oil. When the oil is hot, add the cakes and cook until golden brown, 2 to 3 minutes per side. (Don't crowd the skillet; you might have to do more than one batch.) Serve immediately drizzled with Remoulade Sauce.

REMOULADE SAUCE

Makes about 1 cup

1 cup vegan mayonnaise

2 tablespoons lemon juice

2 tablespoons finely chopped chives

1 tablespoon Dijon mustard

1 tablespoon prepared horseradish

1 tablespoon tomato paste

1 tablespoon sweet paprika

½ teaspoon fine sea salt

¼ teaspoon white pepper

In a medium bowl, whisk together the mayonnaise, lemon juice, chives, mustard, horseradish, tomato paste, paprika, salt, and pepper. Set aside in the refrigerator until ready to serve.

Serve the cakes on a simple mixed green salad dressed with a lemony vinaigrette.

Garlicky White Bean Spread on Crostini

**_Makes about 40 bite-sized
appetizers_**

1 (15-ounce) can cannellini beans,
   drained

2 to 4 cloves garlic

3 tablespoons lemon juice

1 tablespoon extra virgin olive oil

$\frac{1}{4}$ teaspoon fine sea salt,
   or more to taste

$\frac{1}{8}$ teaspoon pepper

2 teaspoons chopped fresh Italian
   parsley, basil, or a combination

Additional chopped fresh Italian
   parsley or basil, or diced roasted
   red peppers, for garnish (optional)

About 40 crostini, homemade
   (recipe follows) or store bought

In the bowl of a food processor, combine the beans, 2 cloves of garlic, lemon juice, olive oil, salt, and pepper. Puree, stopping to scrape the bowl as needed. Taste and add more garlic or salt as desired. Stir in the 2 teaspoons of chopped parsley and/or basil.

Top each crostini with about 2 teaspoons of the bean spread. Top the spread with a sprinkle of chopped herbs or a couple of pieces of diced peppers, if desired. Arrange crostini on a platter and serve.

If you don't feel like laboring over 40 appetizers, serve the bean spread in a bowl and arrange the crostini alongside.

CROSTINI

Makes 40 crostini

10 slices whole wheat bread
   or 1 baguette
Refined coconut oil,
   melted (optional)

Preheat oven to 350°F.

If using bread, trim off the crusts and cut each slice into quarters. If using a baguette, cut it diagonally into about 20 slices, then cut each slice in half. Brush the bread with the coconut oil, if desired.

Arrange the bread in a single layer on 1 or 2 large rimmed baking sheets. Bake for 8 to 15 minutes, depending on the bread, until dry and slightly browned. Cool before using.

Herbed "Egg" Salad Scoops

Makes about 40 appetizers

5 large heads endive

14 to 16 ounces extra firm tofu,
   drained and pressed (to squeeze
   out excess water)

¼ small diced white onion
   (about ¼ cup)

¼ cup vegan mayonnaise

1 tablespoon Dijon mustard

1½ tablespoons lemon juice

1 teaspoon fine sea salt

¼ teaspoon white pepper

¼ teaspoon curry powder

1 tablespoon chopped fresh chives

1 tablespoon chopped fresh parsley

2 teaspoons chopped fresh tarragon

Separate the endive leaves, setting aside about 40 (reserve the rest for another use).

In a large bowl, crumble the tofu. Stir in the onion, mayonnaise, mustard, lemon juice, salt, pepper, and curry powder. Add about 2 teaspoons of the chives, about 2 teaspoons of the parsley, and about 1 teaspoon of the tarragon.

About 1 tablespoon at a time, place a scoop of salad onto the tip of each endive leaf. Arrange the leaves on a platter, sprinkle with the remaining herbs, and serve.

Mock Chopped Liver

Makes about 2 cups

2 tablespoons refined coconut oil

1 onion, cut into rough ½-inch dice

1 pound cremini (brown)
  mushrooms, thickly sliced

3 cloves garlic, roughly chopped

1 cup raw cashews, toasted

2 tablespoons nut oil, such as
  walnut or hazelnut, or extra
  virgin olive oil

1 tablespoon Bragg's Liquid
  Aminos, or more to taste (or two
  teaspoons tamari or soy sauce)

1 teaspoon fine sea salt,
  or more to taste

¼ teaspoon pepper, or more to taste

Heat the coconut oil in a large skillet over medium-high. Add the onions and cook, stirring occasionally, until they just begin to brown, about 3 minutes. Add the mushrooms and cook, stirring occasionally, until the mushrooms are limp and the released liquid has almost entirely evaporated, 8 to 10 minutes. Stir in the garlic and cook for 1 minute. Set aside to cool.

In a food processor, pulse the cashews until finely chopped. Add the mushroom mixture, nut oil, Bragg's Liquid Aminos, salt, and pepper and process until smooth. Add more Bragg's Liquid Aminos, salt, and/or pepper to taste.

It's good enough to eat with a spoon, but serve it on crackers or something. Be a lady.

Spicy Mixed Nuts

Makes about 3 cups

1½ teaspoons Ener-G egg replacer

2 tablespoons warm water

1 pound roasted, salted mixed nuts

⅓ cup evaporated cane sugar

2 teaspoons kosher
or other coarse salt

1½ teaspoons cayenne powder

Do not eat entire batch in one sitting. Seriously.

Preheat oven to 250°F.

In a medium bowl, whisk the egg replacer and water until foamy. Add the nuts and toss to coat. Transfer the nuts to a strainer and let drain for at least 2 minutes.

Meanwhile, wipe out the bowl and combine the sugar, salt, and cayenne. Add the nuts, tossing to coat. Spread the nuts in a single layer on a large rimmed baking sheet. Bake for 40 minutes. Stir with a spatula and spread the nuts out again. Reduce the oven to 200°F and bake another 30 minutes, or until dry. The nuts will crisp as they cool to room temperature. Thoroughly cooled, they can be stored for up to one week in an airtight container.

Stuffed Mushrooms

Makes 20 mushrooms

2 tablespoons refined coconut oil,
   plus more for greasing baking sheet

20 large (2 to 2 ½ inches across)
   white mushrooms

1 red bell pepper, finely diced

1 shallot, finely diced

½ teaspoon dried oregano

6 tablespoons whole wheat
   seasoned or Italian bread crumbs

6 tablespoons vegan
   Parmesan cheese

¼ cup chopped fresh Italian parsley

1 teaspoon fine sea salt

½ teaspoon pepper

Preheat oven to 400°F. Grease a large, rimmed baking sheet.

Carefully pull the stems from the mushroom caps; set stems aside. Arrange the caps, stem sides down, on the prepared baking sheet and bake until they leak liquid, about 10 minutes. Remove from the oven and set aside.

While the caps are baking, finely chop the stems. Heat the oil in a large skillet over medium-high. Add the stems and cook, stirring occasionally, until golden brown, 2 to 3 minutes. Add the bell pepper, shallot, and oregano and cook, stirring occasionally, until the bell pepper is tender, about 3 minutes. Transfer the mixture to a medium bowl to cool slightly, then stir in the bread crumbs, cheese, parsley, salt, and pepper.

Turn the mushroom caps over and spoon in the filling, pressing gently and slightly mounding it. Bake until the mushrooms are tender and the stuffing is browned, about 20 minutes. Then eat every last one before anyone else can try them.

Spicy Sushi Rolls with Avocado and Cucumber

> If you're short on patience or easily frustrated, you're better off going to your local Japanese restaurant. There is a Zen art to making sushi rolls, and if you're cursing and screaming and carrying on, your sushi will sucky.

Makes 4 rolls

¼ cup vegan mayonnaise

½ to 1 tablespoon sriracha
(or other chili sauce; see note),
or more to taste

4 sheets nori (see note)

About 3 cups prepared Brown
Sushi Rice (recipe follows)

1 avocado, peeled, pitted, and sliced

½ small cucumber, peeled, halved
lengthwise, seeded, and sliced
lengthwise

½ small carrot, julienned

Soy sauce for serving

Wasabi paste for serving (see note)

Pickled ginger for serving (see note)

Special equipment:
bamboo sushi mat (see note)

In a small bowl, combine the mayonnaise with ½ tablespoon of sriracha. Taste and add more sriracha if you like.

Place a bamboo sushi mat on a clean work surface, with the sticks in the mat parallel to you. Place a sheet of nori on the mat, shiny side down, shorter edge toward you. Have a shallow bowl of water nearby. Dampen your hands in the water, shaking off the excess moisture. Use your fingers to press about ⅔ cup of Sushi Rice onto the nori, covering ⅔ of the sheet closest to you (if the rice sticks to your hands as you work, redampen them in the water). Drizzle about 1 tablespoon of the mayonnaise mixture on top of the rice in a line parallel to you, about

1 inch in from closest edge. Top the mayonnaise with ¼ of the avocado, ¼ of the cucumber, and ¼ of the carrots.

Take a deep breath and smile. Holding the fillings firmly in place with the fingertips of both hands, use both thumbs to lift the edge of the mat closest to you up and over, enclosing the fillings. Squeeze gently to make a compact roll. Raise the end of the mat slightly to avoid rolling it in with the nori, and continue rolling, squeezing occasionally, until the sushi is completely rolled in to a tight cylinder. If necessary, dampen the end of the nori to help it seal, then allow the roll to sit for a minute or two. Slice the roll into 8 pieces with a sharp, lightly moistened knife. Repeat with the remaining ingredients, making 4 rolls total. Serve the sushi on a platter with soy sauce, wasabi, and pickled ginger.

SRIRACHA (an Asian chili sauce), NORI (seaweed sheets), WASABI paste, and PICKLED GINGER can be found in the Asian section of most major supermarkets.

Look for a BAMBOO SUSHI MAT there, too, or in the utensils section, or at cookware stores. Before you start, cover the sushi mat with plastic wrap to make it easy to clean.

Brown Sushi Rice

Makes about 3 cups

1 cup short-grain brown rice
   (see note)

2 cups water

3 tablespoons seasoned
   rice vinegar (see note)

Sushi rice is traditionally made with white rice, but we're health rebels!

Seasoned rice vinegar can be found in the Asian section of most major supermarkets.

In a 2-quart saucepan over high heat, combine the rice and water. Bring to a boil, reduce the heat to a simmer, cover, and cook until the water is absorbed and the rice is tender, about 45 minutes. Remove from the heat and let the rice stand, covered, at least 10 minutes.

Turn the cooked rice out into a large shallow bowl or dish. Use a rice paddle or spatula and a slashing motion to spread the rice evenly in the bowl (don't toss; the rice can get gummy). Drizzle the rice vinegar over the rice. With the same slashing motion, mix until the grains are coated and glossy. Cover with a damp kitchen towel and cool at room temperature until cool enough to handle (do not refrigerate). Once cool, the rice will remain the right texture for making sushi for several hours.

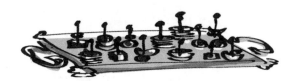

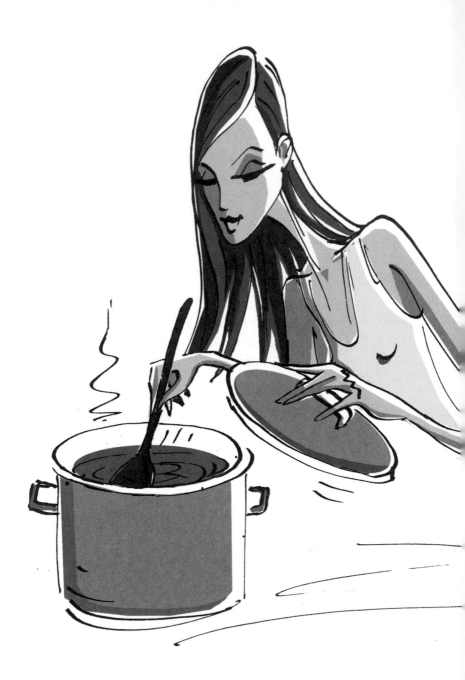

Sassy Soups
AND STEWS

We like soup. There. We said it.
Don't think that makes us boring old farts.
These soups are really friggin' good. And
you can make a big batch and just heat it up for
dinner a few nights in a row. More time for sex!
Hah! Who's a boring old fart now, bitch?

Cheezy Cream of Broccoli

"Chicken" Noodle

Lentil Vegetable

Split Pea

Red Wine "Beef" Stew

Super Easy Creamy
"Chicken" and Gravy Stew

Cheezy Cream of Broccoli Soup

Makes about 7 cups

1 tablespoon refined coconut oil

1 onion, diced

4 cups roughly chopped
broccoli florets

2 teaspoons fine sea salt

1 teaspoon pepper

1½ cups low-sodium
vegetable stock

4 cups soy or rice milk

¼ cup arrowroot (or 5 tablespoons
cornstarch) dissolved in ¼ cup
cold water

6 ounces vegan cheddar cheese

So. Friggin'. Good.

Heat the coconut oil in a 4- to 6-quart stockpot over medium heat. Add the onion and cook, stirring occasionally, for 2 minutes. Add the broccoli, salt, and pepper and cook, stirring occasionally, until the onion is translucent and the broccoli is crisp-tender, about 4 minutes.

Stir in the stock, increase the heat to high, bring to a boil, and reduce the heat to a simmer. Cook until the broccoli is very tender, about 10 minutes. Remove from the heat and stir in about 1 cup of the soy or rice milk.

Transfer the mixture to a blender. On low or medium speed, puree until smooth. Transfer the mixture back to the pot, return to medium high heat, and stir in the remaining soy milk. When the soup returns to a simmer, add the arrowroot mixture and cheese, stirring until the cheese melts.

"Chicken" Noodle Soup

Just like mom used to make—minus the pieces of decomposing, rotting chicken carcass.

Makes about 9 cups

1 tablespoon refined coconut oil

1 carrot, halved lengthwise and
   cut into ¼-inch slices

1 celery stalk, cut into ¼-inch slices

½ onion, cut into ½-inch dice

4 ounces white or cremini (brown)
   mushrooms, cut into ¼-inch slices

1 teaspoon fine sea salt

½ teaspoon pepper

¼ teaspoon curry powder

1 bay leaf

8 cups vegan chicken stock (hot water
   mixed with vegan chicken bouillon
   according to package directions)

2 teaspoons Bragg's Liquid Aminos (or
   1¼ teaspoons tamari or soy sauce)

8 ounces vegan chicken strips or
   chunks (if frozen, no need to thaw)

4 ounces whole wheat or
   brown rice pasta

Heat the coconut oil in a 4- to 6-quart stockpot over medium heat. Add the carrot, celery, and onion and cook, stirring occasionally, until crisp tender, about 2 minutes. Add the mushrooms, salt, pepper, and curry powder and cook until the mushrooms release their juices, about 2 minutes.

Stir in the stock, Bragg's Liquid Aminos, and bay leaf. Increase the heat to high and bring to a boil. Add the chicken and pasta. When the soup returns to a boil, reduce to a simmer. Cook until the pasta is tender (time will depend on type of pasta). Remove the bay leaf and serve.

Lentil Vegetable Soup

Makes about 8 cups

1 tablespoon refined coconut oil

½ red bell pepper, cut into ½-inch dice

½ yellow bell pepper,
   cut into ½-inch dice

½ onion, cut into ½-inch dice

1 zucchini, quartered lengthwise
   and cut into ½-inch slices

1 yellow squash, quartered lengthwise and cut into ½-inch slices

4 cloves garlic, minced

1 teaspoon fine sea salt

½ teaspoon pepper

½ teaspoon dried marjoram

½ teaspoon dried thyme

⅛ teaspoon cayenne powder

6 cups low-sodium vegetable stock

1½ cups lentils

1 tablespoon tamari or soy sauce

½ teaspoon sesame oil

1 14.5-ounce can diced tomatoes
   (with juices)

Heat the coconut oil in a 4- to 6-quart stockpot over medium heat. Add the red bell pepper, yellow bell pepper, and onion and cook, stirring occasionally, for 2 minutes. Add the zucchini, yellow squash, garlic, salt, pepper, marjoram, thyme, and cayenne and cook, stirring occasionally, for 1 minute.

Stir in the stock, lentils, and tamari or soy sauce. Increase the heat to high, bring to a boil, and reduce to a simmer. Cook until the lentils are tender, about 30 minutes. Add the sesame oil and tomatoes, stirring until the tomatoes are heated through.

WARNING: Lentils make you toot for hours. Plan accordingly.

Split Pea Soup

Makes about 8 cups

1 tablespoon refined
coconut or safflower oil

8 strips vegan bacon,
cut into ¼-inch dice

1 onion, cut into ¼-inch dice

4 cloves garlic, minced

1½ teaspoons dried oregano

1½ teaspoons fine sea salt

¾ teaspoon pepper

10 cups vegan chicken stock (hot
water mixed with vegan chicken
bouillon according to package
directions)

3 cups split peas

1 carrot, cut into ¼-inch dice

1 celery stalk, cut into ¼-inch dice

Heat the oil in a 4- to 6-quart stockpot over medium, Add the bacon and cook, stirring occasionally, for 2 minutes. Add the onion and cook, stirring occasionally, for 1 minute. Add the garlic, oregano, salt, and pepper and cook, stirring occasionally, for 1 minute.

Stir in the stock and split peas. Increase the heat to high, bring to a boil, and reduce to a simmer. Cook for 45 minutes, stirring occasionally. Add the carrots and celery and cook, stirring occasionally, another 20 minutes, or until the carrots and celery are tender and the soup is the desired thickness.

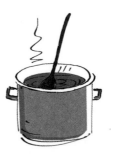

Red Wine "Beef" Stew

Serves 6

½ cup whole wheat pastry flour

1 tablespoon minced fresh rosemary

1 teaspoon fine sea salt

½ teaspoon pepper

12 ounces vegan beef strips
    or chunks (thawed, if frozen)

1 tablespoon refined coconut oil

4 cloves garlic, minced

4½ cups low-sodium
    vegetable stock

1½ cups dry red wine

3 carrots, cut into 1-inch chunks

1 pound red potatoes, cut into
    1-inch chunks

1 onion, cut into 1-inch chunks

½ pounds cremini (brown) mush-
    rooms, halved (or quartered if large)

1 cup fresh or frozen peas

In a medium bowl, combine the flour, rosemary, salt, and pepper. Add the beef and toss to coat.

Heat the coconut oil in a 4- to 6-quart stockpot over medium heat. Add the beef mixture and cook, stirring occasionally, for 5 minutes. Add the garlic and cook, stirring occasionally, for 1 minute.

Stir in the stock, wine, and carrots. Increase the heat to high, bring to a boil, and reduce to a simmer. Cook for 15 minutes, stirring occasionally. Add the potato and onion and cook, stirring occasionally, for 15 minutes. Add the mushrooms and cook, stirring occasionally, for 15 minutes. Add the peas, stirring until the peas are heated through.

And you thought you needed a dead animal to make your stew hearty... Shame on you!

Super Easy Creamy "Chicken" and Gravy Stew

Serves 6

4 cups quadruple-strength vegan chicken stock (hot water mixed with four times the vegan chicken bouillon indicated on package directions)

1 (12-ounce) container vegan sour cream

¼ cup arrowroot or 5 tablespoons corn starch dissolved in ¼ cup water

¼ cup coarse nutritional yeast

2 teaspoons Bragg's Liquid Aminos (or 1¼ teaspoons tamari or soy sauce)

1½ teaspoons garlic powder

1½ teaspoons onion powder

1 teaspoon dried tarragon

1 teaspoon fine sea salt

½ teaspoon pepper

½ teaspoon turmeric

16 ounces vegan chicken strips or chunks (if frozen, no need to thaw)

2 (14-ounce bags) frozen mixed vegetables, whatever vegetables you like — big chunks work best

In a 4- to 6-quart stockpot over medium high, combine the stock, sour cream, arrowroot mixture, nutritional yeast, Bragg's Liquid Aminos, garlic powder, onion powder, tarragon, salt, pepper, and turmeric, whisking until smooth. Bring the mixture to a simmer and stir in the chicken and vegetables. Return to a simmer and cook, stirring occasionally, until the chicken and vegetables are heated through (time will depend on the size of the chicken and vegetable pieces).

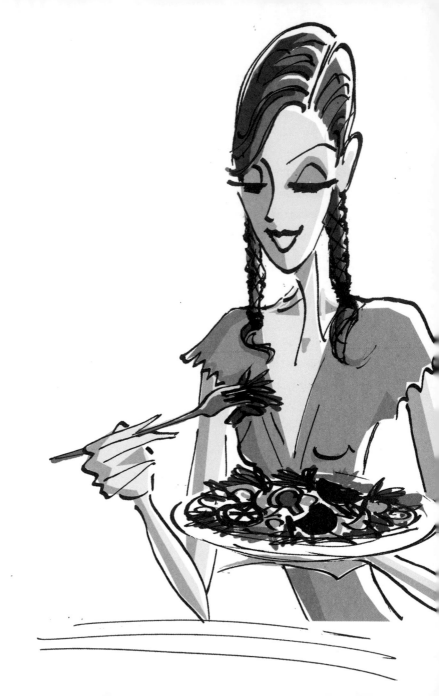

Skinny-Ass
SALADS

Let's face it: Salads can be so fucking lame.
But they're really good for our bodies
(especially for pooping), so we gotta have 'em.
We crafted these little green monsters to be healthy
and yummy. This way, we don't have to suffer
through salads. We can actually enjoy them.

Caesar Salad with
Homemade Herbed Croutons

Greek Salad

Chef's Salad

Tabouleh

Potato Salad with Fresh Dill

Edamame Three-bean Salad

Creamy Cole Slaw

Mediterranean Pasta Salad

Caesar Salad with Homemade Herbed Croutons

Serves 6 as an entree

or 8 to 10 as an appetizer

3 slices vegan whole wheat
  bread, diced

2 tablespoons refined coconut oil,
  melted, or safflower oil

1 teaspoon herbes de Provence
  (see note)

½ teaspoon fine sea salt

3 heads romaine lettuce,
  cut or torn into bite-sized pieces

About 1½ cups Vegan Caesar
  Dressing (see page 154)

Preheat oven to 375°F.

In a large bowl, combine the bread and oil. Stir in the herbes de Provence and salt. Spread the mixture onto a rimmed baking sheet and bake for 10 minutes. Remove from the oven and toss. Bake for 5 minutes more, or until browned. Cool the croutons thoroughly before using (or storing in an airtight container for up to 1 week).

In a large bowl, combine the romaine with the Vegan Caesar Dressing to taste. Toss in the croutons and serve.

> **HERBES de PROVENCE**
> is a dried herb blend. If you can't find it at your supermarket, try a specialty food store or substitute dried sage, thyme, rosemary, marjoram, or a combination.

Greek Salad

Serves 6 to 8 as a side dish

or 4 as an entree

2 tablespoons red wine vinegar

4 garlic cloves, minced

1 teaspoon Dijon mustard

½ teaspoon fine sea salt

½ teaspoon pepper

¼ cup extra virgin olive oil

2 tomatoes, cut into ¾-inch dice

1 cucumber, peeled, halved lengthwise, and cut into ¼-inch slices

½ cup pitted black olives,
   preferably Kalamata

¼ red onion, thinly sliced

3 cups Marinated Tofu "Feta"
   (see page 159)

Salad greens (optional)

In a small bowl, whisk together the red wine vinegar, garlic, mustard, salt, and pepper. Slowly whisk in the olive oil; set the dressing aside.

In a large bowl, combine the tomatoes, cucumber, olives, and onion. Gently toss in the Marinated Tofu "Feta" and dressing to taste. Serve as is for a side dish, or on top of salad greens for an entree.

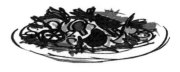

Chef's Salad

Serves 4 as an entree

1 head red leaf, green leaf, or
  iceberg lettuce, torn into
  bite-sized pieces

4 slices vegan cheddar cheese,
  cut into strips

4 slices vegan Swiss or American
  cheese, cut into strips

4 slices vegan ham, cut into strips

4 slices vegan turkey, cut into strips

4 Roma tomatoes, cut into wedges

½ to 1 cup salad dressing of your
  choice (For Ranch see page 151,
  Thousand Island page 152,
  Caesar page 154)

1¼ cups "Egg" Salad (see page 44)

2 tablespoons chopped Italian
  parsley, for garnish (optional)

Arrange the lettuce on 4 plates, dividing it evenly. Artfully arrange the cheeses, ham, turkey, and tomatoes on top, dividing them evenly. Drizzle the salad dressing over the salads. Top with "Egg" Salad, dividing it evenly, and sprinkle with parsley, if using. Serve immediately.

Tabouleh

Serves 6 to 8

¾ cup bulgur wheat (see note)

1 cup boiling water

¼ cup extra virgin olive oil

1½ tablespoons lemon juice

½ teaspoon fine sea salt

¼ teaspoon pepper

1 tomato, cut into ½-inch dice

½ cucumber, peeled and cut
   into ½-inch dice

¼ red onion, cut into ½-inch dice

⅓ cup roughly chopped fresh parsley

⅓ cup roughly chopped fresh mint

In a large bowl, combine the bulgur wheat and boiling water. Cover and set aside for 30 minutes. Meanwhile, in a small bowl, combine the olive oil, lemon juice, salt, and pepper; set aside.

Add the tomato, cucumber, and onion to the bulgur wheat. Stir in the parsley and mint. Add the dressing and toss gently.

> **BULGUR WHEAT** can be found in the bulk section of many major supermarkets as well as at natural food stores.

Potato Salad with Fresh Dill

Serves 6 to 8

6 cups water

1½ pounds red or Yukon gold
   potatoes, cut into 1-inch cubes

About 2½ teaspoons fine sea salt

⅓ cup vegan mayonnaise

¼ cup sweet pickle relish

1 teaspoon white wine vinegar

¼ teaspoon pepper

1 celery stalk, cut into ½-inch dice
   or thinly sliced

2 scallions, thinly sliced

2 tablespoons chopped fresh dill

In a 3- or 4-quart stockpot, combine the water with about 2 teaspoons of the salt. Add the potatoes and place the pot over high heat. Bring to a boil, reduce to a simmer, and cook until the potatoes are tender, about 5 minutes. Strain the potatoes and transfer them to a large bowl to cool.

Meanwhile, in a small bowl, whisk together the mayonnaise, pickle relish, vinegar, pepper, and remaining ½ teaspoon of salt.

When the potatoes are cool, gently toss in the celery, scallions, and dill. Add the mayonnaise mixture and gently toss.

Edamame Three-bean Salad

Serves 6 to 8

2 tablespoons red wine vinegar

1 teaspoon Dijon mustard

½ teaspoon fine sea salt

¼ teaspoon pepper

3 tablespoons extra virgin olive oil

1 ear corn or ½ cup frozen corn
(rinsed under cold water to thaw)

1 cup shelled soy beans (edamame)
(see note)

1 (15- to 16-ounce) can red kidney
beans, drained and rinsed

1 (15- to 16-ounce) can garbanzo
beans, drained and rinsed

2 scallions, cut into ½-inch slices

½ red bell pepper,
cut into ½-inch dice

2 tablespoons chopped fresh
Italian parsley

2 tablespoons chopped fresh
cilantro, basil, or a combination

In a small bowl, whisk together the red wine vinegar, mustard, salt, and pepper. Slowly whisk in the olive oil; set aside.

Cut the kernels off the ear of corn and place them in a large bowl. Stir in the soy beans, kidney beans, garbanzo beans, scallions, bell pepper, parsley, and cilantro and/or basil. Gently toss in the dressing.

SHELLED SOY BEANS, also known as edamame, can be found in the produce or freezer section of many major supermarkets, as well as at natural and Asian food stores. If frozen, rinse under cold water to thaw.

Creamy Cole Slaw

Serves 4 to 6

¼ cup vegan mayonnaise

¼ cup vegan sour cream

½ tablespoon white wine vinegar

½ tablespoon agave nectar

½ teaspoon fine sea salt

½ head green cabbage, quartered, cored, and thinly shredded

⅛ small red cabbage, halved, cored and thinly shredded

1 carrot, shredded

In a small bowl, whisk together the mayonnaise, sour cream, vinegar, agave nectar, and salt; set aside.

In a large bowl, combine the green cabbage, red cabbage, and carrot. Add the dressing and toss until well combined. Cover and refrigerate for 24 to 48 hours to let the flavors develop.

Lazy bitches can replace the green cabbage, red cabbage, and carrot with a one-pound bag of prepared slaw mix.

Mediterranean Pasta Salad

Serves 10 to 12

3 quarts water

About 1½ tablespoons fine sea salt

1 pound whole wheat fusilli, rotelli,
  or other shaped pasta

½ cup oil-packed julienned
  sun-dried tomatoes, drained
  (save 2 tablespoons of oil)

1 lemon

1 (14.75-ounce) jar marinated
  artichoke hearts, drained (save
  2 tablespoons of marinade)

½ cup pitted black olives (Kalamata,
  Niçoise — anything other than
  canned Mission olives)

½ cup chopped fresh basil

In a 4- to 6-quart stockpot over high heat, combine the water and salt. Bring the water to a boil, add the pasta, and cook according to the package directions. When the pasta is done, drain it (don't rinse it), transfer it to a large bowl, and toss with the 2 tablespoons of reserved sun dried tomato oil. Set aside to cool.

Meanwhile, juice the lemon into a small bowl. Whisk in the 2 tablespoons of artichoke marinade. Set aside.

When the pasta is cool, gently toss in the marinade mixture. Cut the artichoke pieces in half (or quarters if large) and add them to the pasta, along with the sun-dried tomatoes, olives, and basil. Gently toss to combine. Serve immediately or refrigerate until serving.

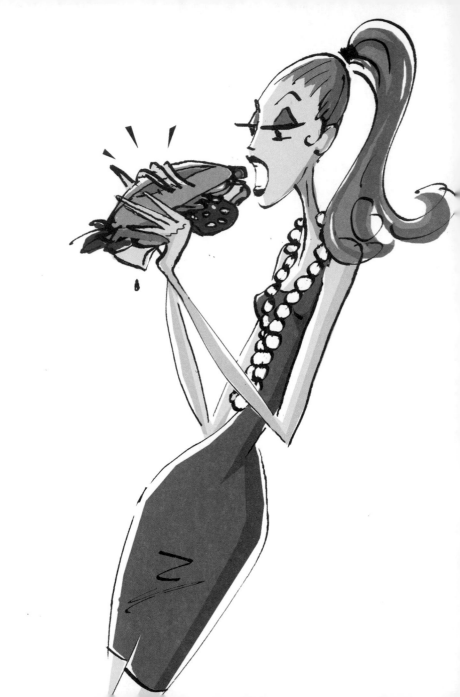

Hearty-Ass
SANDWICHES

*The only thing better than pigging out on
a big-ass sandwich? Getting seconds from off
your own face. Moo! Chow down, cowgirls!*

Club Sandwich

Reuben-esque

"Tuna" Salad

"Chicken" Salad

Philly "Cheesesteak"

Veggie Burger

"Chicken" Panini

Club Sandwich

Makes 4 sandwiches

8 slices vegan whole wheat
   bread, toasted

About 3 tablespoons
   vegan mayonnaise

1 avocado, sliced

8 ounces vegan turkey
   or chicken slices

2 tomatoes, sliced

12 strips vegan bacon

4 large lettuce leaves

Spread each slice of toast with about 2 teaspoons of the mayonnaise. Top the mayonnaise side with 4 slices with avocado, turkey or chicken, tomatoes, bacon, and lettuce, dividing the ingredients evenly. Top with remaining toast, mayonnaise side down.

Reuben-esque

....

Makes 1 sandwich

¼ cup low-sodium vegetable stock

1 teaspoon garlic powder

½ teaspoon Bragg's Liquid Aminos
   (or ¼ teaspoon tamari or soy sauce)

6 to 12 strips vegan bacon

2 slices vegan whole wheat rye
   bread, toasted

2 slices vegan Swiss cheese

¼ cup drained sauerkraut

2 tablespoons Thousand Island
   Dressing (see page 152)

Preheat broiler.

In a 12-inch nonstick skillet over medium heat, combine the stock, garlic powder, and Bragg's Liquid Aminos. When the mixture begins simmering, add the bacon strips, spreading them out evenly. Cook until the liquid has evaporated, about 2 minutes. Turn and cook the other side until the garlic powder begins to brown, about 1 minute.

Remove from heat; set aside.

Arrange the bacon on top of one slice of toast. Top with the cheese and place on a baking sheet. Arrange the sauerkraut on the other slice of toast and place on the baking sheet. Place the baking sheet under the broiler until the cheese melts and the sauerkraut is warm. (Time will depend on the cheese. Keep a watchful eye on it! It could only take a minute or so.) Remove from the broiler, top sauerkraut with Thousand Island Dressing, and sandwich the two toasts together. Cut in half and serve.

FYI: Six slices of bacon strips make for a satisfying sandwich; twelve make for a whaler. For the complete deli experience, hold the sandwich together with toothpicks and serve a sour pickle on the side.

"Tuna" Salad Sandwich

Makes 3 or 4 sandwiches

2 cups finely shredded parsnip

1 celery stalk, finely diced

¼ small red or white onion,

   finely diced

1 lemon

¼ cup vegan mayonnaise

½ tablespoon sweet pickle relish

1 teaspoon coarse nutritional yeast

½ teaspoon kelp powder

¼ teaspoon fine sea salt

6 to 8 slices vegan

   whole wheat bread

In a large bowl, combine the parsnip, celery, and onion. Zest, then halve the lemon. Add the lemon zest and juice from one half (save the other for another use) to the parsnip mixture, along with the mayonnaise, relish, yeast, kelp powder, and salt, stirring to combine.

Spread the tuna salad on 3 or 4 slices of bread, top with remaining 3 or 4 slices, and serve.

"Chicken" Salad Sandwich

Makes 3 or 4 sandwiches

½ cup vegan mayonnaise

2 teaspoons lemon juice

1 tablespoon coarse nutritional yeast

½ tablespoon agave nectar

¼ teaspoon fine sea salt

¼ teaspoon curry powder

⅛ teaspoon pepper

2 cups chopped or shredded vegan
  chicken strips or chunks (thawed,
  if frozen)

¼ cup halved (quartered if large)
  seedless red grapes (optional)

1 celery stalk, finely diced

¼ small red or white onion,
  finely diced

2 tablespoons chopped fresh
  Italian parsley

6 to 8 slices vegan
  whole wheat bread

In a small bowl, combine the mayonnaise, lemon juice, yeast, agave nectar, salt, curry powder, and pepper. In a large bowl, combine the chicken, grapes (if using), celery, onion, and parsley. Add the mayonnaise mixture to the chicken mixture, tossing gently.

Spread the chicken salad on 3 or 4 slices of bread, top with remaining 3 or 4 slices, and serve.

If you're one of those lunatics who doesn't eat bread, you can also serve this salad on a bed of lettuce.

Philly "Cheesesteak"

Makes 2 sandwiches

2 tablespoons refined coconut oil

½ red bell pepper,
cut into ¼-inch slices

½ yellow or green bell pepper, cut
into ¼-inch slices

½ red onion, cut into ¼-inch slices

4 ounces brown or white
mushrooms, sliced

2 cloves garlic, minced

½ teaspoon fine sea salt

¼ teaspoon pepper

12 slices vegan bacon

About ¼ cup water

4 slices vegan American cheese

2 vegan soft whole wheat rolls

Heat the coconut oil in a 10- to 12-inch skillet over medium heat. Add the peppers and cook, stirring occasionally, for 5 minutes. Add the onion and cook, stirring occasionally, until onion is lightly browned, about 3 minutes. Add the mushrooms and cook, stirring occasionally, for 3 minutes more. Add the garlic, reduce the heat to low, and cook, stirring occasionally, until all the vegetables are very tender, 5 to 7 minutes. Remove from the heat and stir in the salt and pepper. Transfer to a bowl, cover with a dish or plastic wrap, and set aside to steam.

Return the skillet to medium heat and add about 2 tablespoons of water. Use a spatula to loosen any caramelized bits in the skillet, then add the bacon (it can overlap slightly, but you may have to do two batches). Cook about 2 minutes, turning once. If the skillet gets dry, add more water, 1 tablespoon at a time (you want the bacon tender and juicy, not crisp).

Cut the rolls almost in half lengthwise, then gently fold each open. Pile 6 strips of bacon, 2 slices of cheese, and half of the veggies onto each of the rolls.

Veggie Burger Four Ways

Funny how we associate being "All-American" with eating the flesh of a tortured, slaughtered animal … Well, not in Skinny Bitch world!

ALL-AMERICAN BASIC BURGER

Makes 4 burgers

4 vegan burger patties

4 slices vegan cheese (optional)

4 large lettuce leaves

1 large tomato,
   cut into 4 thick slices

4 thin slices red onion

12 slices "bread and butter" pickles

4 vegan whole wheat hamburger
   buns, split and toasted

Mustard, ketchup, and vegan
   mayonnaise, for serving

Grill or pan-sauté the burger patties according to package directions. If using cheese, top each patty with one slice of cheese during the last minute of cooking.

Meanwhile, arrange lettuce, tomato, red onion, and pickles on serving plates, dividing evenly. When the patties are done, sandwich one between each bun, arrange on plates, and serve.

PIZZA BURGER

Makes 4 burgers

4 vegan burger patties

4 slices vegan mozzarella cheese

16 slices vegan pepperoni

4 vegan whole wheat hamburger

buns, split and toasted

¾ cup Pizza Sauce (see page 157),

warmed

12 large basil leaves,

cut into thin strips

Pan-sauté the burger patties according to package directions. Top each patty with one slice of cheese during the last minute of cooking. Add the pepperoni to the pan during the last minute as well, just to warm it.

Place one cooked patty on the bottom of each bun. Top with Pizza Sauce, pepperoni, and basil leaves, dividing evenly. Serve immediately.

CALIFORNIA BURGER

Makes 4 burgers

4 vegan burger patties

4 vegan whole wheat hamburger

buns, split and toasted

1 avocado, sliced

1 cup loosely packed alfalfa sprouts

½ cup Thousand Island Dressing

(see page 152)

Grill or pan-sauté the burger patties according to package directions. Place one cooked patty on the bottom of each bun. Top with avocado, sprouts, and Thousand Island Dressing, dividing evenly. Serve immediately.

BACON AND CARAMELIZED ONION CHEESEBURGERS WITH AGAVE-DIJON

Makes 4 burgers

¼ cup refined coconut oil

2 large yellow onions,
   cut into ¼-inch slices

¼ teaspoon fine sea salt

⅛ teaspoon pepper

2 tablespoons agave nectar

2 tablespoons Dijon mustard

8 slices vegan bacon

4 vegan burger patties

4 slices vegan cheese

4 vegan whole wheat hamburger
   buns, split and toasted

Heat the coconut oil in a large skillet over medium-high heat. Add the onions and cook, stirring occasionally, until translucent, about 5 minutes. Reduce the heat to very low and cook, stirring occasionally, until the onions are deeply golden, about 45 minutes. Stir in the salt and pepper and set aside to cool.

While the onions are cooking, whisk together the agave and mustard in a small bowl; set aside.

While the onions are cooling, cook the bacon according to package directions. Grill or pan-sauté the burger patties according to package directions. Top each patty with one slice of cheese during the last minute of cooking. Place one cooked patty on the bottom of each bun. Top with onions, bacon, and mustard mixture, dividing evenly. Serve immediately.

Grilled "Chicken" Panini Three Ways

"CHICKEN" PARMESAN PANINI

Makes 4 panini

2 tablespoons refined coconut oil
(optional)

4 vegan soft whole wheat rolls or
8 slices vegan whole wheat bread

16 vegan chicken nuggets, cooked
according to package directions

1 cup Basic Red Sauce
(see page 156)

4 to 8 slices vegan
mozzarella cheese

Spread the coconut oil if using, on the top and bottom of the rolls or one side of each slice of bread, dividing it evenly. Cut open the rolls or lay the bread, oiled side down if applicable, on a work surface. Top the bottom half of the rolls or four slices of the bread with the chicken nuggets, Red Sauce, and cheese, dividing evenly.

In a large nonstick skillet over medium heat, cook two sandwiches, covered, about 4 minutes, until golden brown. Flip the sandwiches and cook, uncovered, until the second side is golden brown and the cheese has melted, about 2 minutes. Repeat with the remaining two sandwiches. (Alternately, cook the sandwiches on a panini grill until the bread is golden brown and the cheese has melted, 2 to 3 minutes.)

MEDITERRANEAN "CHICKEN" PANINI

Makes 4 panini

2 tablespoons refined coconut oil (optional)

4 vegan soft whole wheat rolls or 8 slices vegan whole wheat bread

4 vegan chicken patties, cooked according to package directions

About 40 large basil leaves

1 cup roasted red pepper strips, drained

4 to 8 slices vegan mozzarella cheese

Spread the coconut oil, if using, on the top and bottom of the rolls or one side of each slice of bread, dividing it evenly. Cut open the rolls or lay the bread, oiled side down if applicable, on a work surface. Top the bottom half of the rolls or four slices of bread with the chicken, basil, peppers, and cheese, dividing evenly.

In a large nonstick skillet over medium heat, cook two sandwiches, covered, about 4 minutes, until golden brown. Flip the sandwiches and cook, uncovered, until the second side is golden brown and the cheese has melted, about 2 minutes. Repeat with the remaining two sandwiches. (Alternately, cook the sandwiches on a panini grill until the bread is golden brown and the cheese has melted, 2 to 3 minutes.)

BARBECUE "CHICKEN" PANINI

Makes 4 panini

2 tablespoons refined coconut oil
(optional)

4 vegan soft whole wheat rolls or
8 slices vegan whole wheat bread

¾ cup barbecue sauce

4 vegan chicken patties, cooked
according to package directions

1 cup Creamy Cole Slaw
(see page 68)

Spread the coconut oil, if using, on the top and bottom of the rolls or one side of each slice of bread, dividing it evenly. Cut open the rolls or lay the bread, buttered side down if applicable, on a work surface. Top the bottom half of the rolls or four slices of the bread with the barbecue sauce, chicken, and Creamy Cole Slaw, dividing evenly.

In a large nonstick skillet over medium heat, cook two sandwiches, covered, about 4 minutes, until golden brown. Flip the sandwiches and cook, uncovered, until the second side is golden brown, about 2 minutes. Repeat with the remaining two sandwiches. (Alternately, cook the sandwiches on a panini grill until the bread is golden brown, 2 to 3 minutes.)

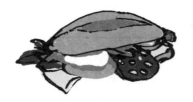

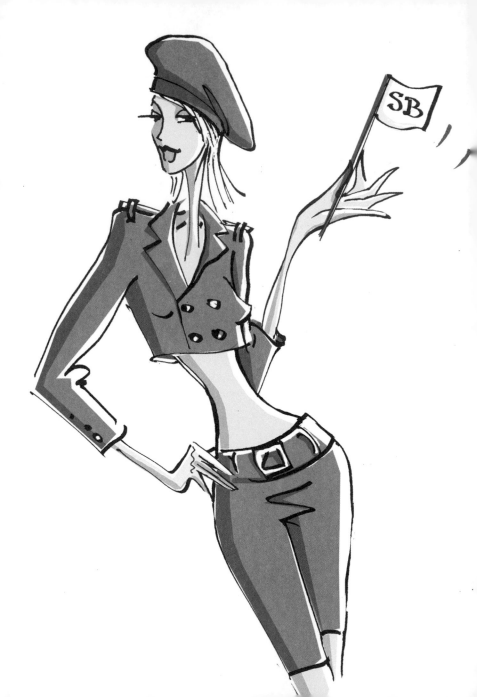

International BITCH

You can totally pretend to be cooler
and worldlier than you actually are.
Just make one of these global goodies.

Falafel

Japanese Soba Noodles
with Steamed Vegetables and Tofu

Potato and Pumpkin Curry
with Brown Basmati Rice

Pad Thai

Veggie Enchiladas

Falafel

Makes 6 sandwiches

1 (15- to 16-ounce) can garbanzo
  beans, drained and rinsed

½ onion, coarsely chopped

2 tablespoons vegan whole wheat
  panko (Japanese bread crumbs)
  or whole wheat bread crumbs

2 tablespoons chickpea
  (garbanzo) flour or whole wheat
  pastry flour

2 tablespoons coarsely chopped
  Italian parsley

½ teaspoon ground cumin

½ teaspoon ground coriander

¼ teaspoon pepper

4 cloves garlic

½ to ¾ teaspoon fine sea salt,
  plus more for sprinkling

About 2 tablespoons refined
  coconut oil, melted, or safflower oil

1 lemon

6 tablespoons tahini

¼ cup water

3 tablespoons extra virgin olive oil

¼ teaspoon paprika

6 (6-inch) pita breads

¼ head iceberg, romaine,
  green leaf, or red leaf lettuce,
  coarsely shredded

1 tomato, cut into thin wedges

½ cucumber, cut into ¼-inch slices

12 to 18 slices dill pickle

Preheat oven to 350°F.

In a food processor, combine the garbanzo beans, onion, panko, flour, parsley, cumin, coriander, pepper, 2 cloves of the garlic, and ½ teaspoon of the salt. Pulse, scraping the sides of the bowl as necessary, to form a coarse paste. Shape the paste into 12 to 14 golf ball-sized rounds. Flatten the balls to about ¾-inch thick and transfer to a rimmed baking sheet. Brush both sides of each ball with the coconut or safflower oil and bake for 45 minutes, turning halfway through, until nicely browned. Set aside to cool.

Meanwhile, juice the lemon. In a small bowl, whisk together the tahini, water, olive oil, paprika, lemon juice, and ¼ teaspoon salt (if using unsalted tahini). Press or finely mince the remaining 2 cloves of garlic and whisk into the tahini sauce. Set aside until ready to serve, or refrigerate for up to a week.

To assemble the sandwiches, cut about 1-inch off the top of each pita, forming a pocket. Add falafel, lettuce, tomato, cucumber, and pickle, dividing evenly. Drizzle each sandwich with about a tablespoon of tahini and pass the rest at the table.

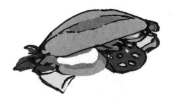

Japanese Soba Noodles with Steamed Vegetables and Tofu

Serves 3 or 4

2 tablespoons mirin (see note)

1 tablespoon minced fresh ginger

1 tablespoon tamari or soy sauce

2 teaspoons sesame oil

¼ cup seasoned rice vinegar

½ pound globe eggplant, cut
   into ½-inch cubes, or Chinese
   or Japanese eggplant, cut into
   ¼-inch slices

About 4¾ teaspoons fine sea salt

8 ounces firm or extra firm tofu,
   cut into ¼-inch cubes

1 carrot, cut into matchsticks

8 ounces buckwheat soba noodles

3 scallions, thinly sliced

1 tablespoon gomasio (see note)
   or toasted sesame seeds

In a large bowl, whisk together the mirin, ginger, tamari or soy sauce, and 1 teaspoon of the sesame oil; set aside.

In a pot fitted with a steamer insert, bring 1 inch of water and 2 tablespoons of the rice vinegar to a boil. Arrange the eggplant in the insert, sprinkle with ¼ teaspoon salt, cover, and steam for 7 minutes. Add the carrot and steam for 5 to 8 minutes. Add the tofu and steam for 3 minutes, until the vegetables are tender and the tofu is heated through.

Meanwhile, in a 4- to 6-quart stockpot, combine 3 quarts of water with about 1½ tablespoons salt. Bring to a boil over high heat, add the noodles, and cook according to package directions until tender. Drain, rinse in cold water, drain again, and return the noodles to the pot. Toss with the remaining 1 teaspoon of sesame oil and cover.

When the vegetable mixture is cooked, add it to the bowl with the mirin mixture, tossing gently.

To serve, place the noodles on plates or a platter and top with the vegetable mixture, scallions, and gomasio, dividing evenly. Serve hot or room temperature.

MIRIN (Japanese rice wine used for cooking) can be found at Asian markets and in the international section of many supermarkets.

GOMASIO is a seasoning made of sesame seeds, seaweed, and sea salt. You can find it at Asian markets and some health food stores.

Potato and Pumpkin Curry with Brown Basmati Rice

Serves 4 to 6

1½ cups brown basmati rice

2½ cups water

¾ teaspoon fine sea salt, divided

2 tablespoons refined coconut oil

1 onion, cut into ¾-inch chunks

2 cloves garlic, minced

1 (14.5-ounce) can diced tomatoes (with juices)

1 cup low-sodium vegetable stock

1 teaspoon ground cumin

1 teaspoon ground coriander

½ teaspoon turmeric

⅛ teaspoon cayenne

⅛ teaspoon ground cinnamon

⅛ teaspoon ground cloves

1 pound red potatoes, cut into ¾-inch chunks

3 cups ¾-inch chunks pumpkin (see note)

1½ tablespoons lemon juice

1 tablespoon chopped fresh cilantro or Italian parsley

In a 2-quart saucepan over high heat, combine the rice, water, and ¼ teaspoon of the salt. Bring to a boil, reduce the heat to a simmer, cover, and cook until the water is absorbed and the rice is tender, about 30 minutes. Remove from the heat and let the rice stand, covered, at least 10 minutes.

While the rice is standing, make the curry: Heat the coconut oil in a 10- to 12-inch skillet over medium high. Add the onion and cook, stirring occasionally, until almost tender, about 3 minutes. Stir in the garlic and cook 1 minute more. Add the tomatoes, stock, cumin, coriander, turmeric, cayenne, cinnamon, cloves, and remaining ½ teaspoon of salt.

Bring to a boil and add the potatoes and pumpkin. Return to a boil, reduce to a simmer, cover, and cook, stirring occasionally, until the potato and pumpkin are tender, about 15 minutes. Remove from heat and stir in lemon juice.

Serve over rice sprinkled with cilantro.

Pumpkin doesn't have to be peeled or skinned before cooking. If you can't find pumpkin, substitute butternut squash, which does have to be skinned. A vegetable peeler works well.

Pad Thai

Serves 3 to 4

6 ounces rice stick noodles

¼ cup agave nectar

¼ cup mirin (see note page 89)

3 tablespoons ketchup

3 tablespoons tamari or soy sauce

1½ tablespoons lime juice

1 tablespoon sriracha (see note
   page 49) or other chili sauce

2 tablespoons refined coconut oil

14 to 16 ounces extra-firm tofu,
   cubed

½ red onion, cut into ¼-inch slices

2 cloves garlic, minced

3 scallions, halved lengthwise and
   cut into 2-inch pieces

2 cups bean sprouts

1 carrot, shredded

¼ cup chopped fresh cilantro, mint,
   or a combination

¼ cup chopped roasted peanuts

4 to 8 lime wedges

Cook the noodles according to package directions. Drain and set aside.

Meanwhile, in a small bowl, whisk together the agave, mirin, ketchup, tamari or soy sauce, lime juice, and sriracha; set aside.

Heat the coconut oil in a 12- to 14-inch wok or skillet over high. Add the tofu and stir-fry for 4 minutes. Add the red onion and stir-fry for 30 seconds. Add the garlic and stir-fry for 30 seconds. Add the noodles and agave nectar mixture and stir-fry until the noodles are softened and evenly coated with sauce. Add the scallions, bean sprouts, and carrot and stir-fry until all the ingredients are well combined and heated through.

Transfer the pad thai to plates or a platter, garnish with cilantro or mint, peanuts and lime wedges, and serve.

We know it seems like the ketchup would crap up the whole dish, but it doesn't. Trust your Bitches.

Veggie Enchiladas

Serves 6

2 tablespoons refined coconut or safflower oil, plus more for frying

1 red bell pepper, cut into ½-inch dice

1 yellow or green bell pepper, cut into ½-inch dice

1 red onion, cut into ½-inch dice

2 cloves garlic, minced

3 cups enchilada sauce, homemade (recipe follows) or canned

1 cup fresh corn, cooked, or frozen corn, thawed

1 (2¼-ounce) can sliced Mission olives, drained

1 teaspoon fine sea salt

½ teaspoon ground cumin

½ teaspoon ground coriander

12 (7-inch) corn tortillas

4 ounces vegan cheddar cheese, shredded

2 scallions, thinly sliced

Preheat oven to 350°F.

Heat 2 tablespoons of the oil in a 10- to 12-inch skillet over medium heat. Add the bell peppers and cook, stirring occasionally, for 5 minutes. Add the onion and cook, stirring occasionally, for 5 minutes. Add the garlic, reduce the heat to low, and cook, stirring occasionally, until all the vegetables are very tender, about 10 minutes. Transfer the vegetables to a large bowl and stir in ½ cup of the enchilada sauce, the corn, olives, salt, cumin, and coriander.

Warm the remaining enchilada sauce in a small saucepan. Then transfer the sauce to a round 8- or 9-inch cake pan. Working one tortilla at a time, use tongs to dip the tortilla into the warm enchilada sauce, dipping to soften the tortilla and coat both sides. Transfer the tortilla to a plate and spoon about ¼ cup of the vegetable mixture down the center of the tortilla. Roll the tortilla into a tight cylinder, enclosing the filling. Transfer the filled tortilla to a 13 x 9-inch baking pan, seam side down. Repeat with remaining tortillas, making 2 rows of 6 enchiladas each in the baking pan.

Pour the leftover dipping sauce over the enchiladas, covering them evenly.

Sprinkle the cheese over the sauce. Bake for 20 minutes, or until the tip of a knife inserted into the center of an enchilada comes out piping hot. Sprinkle with scallions and serve.

....

ENCHILADA SAUCE

Makes about 3 cups

10 dried California or other
    mild chiles, stemmed,
    split, and seeds removed

5 cups water

1 clove garlic

¼ cup refined coconut oil,
    melted, or safflower oil

1 tablespoon tomato paste

1 teaspoon ground cumin

1 teaspoon dried oregano

1 teaspoon fine sea salt

In a 10- to 12-inch skillet over medium high heat, toast the chiles a few at a time until they're blistered and a few shades darker, 1 to 1½ minutes, turning occasionally. Transfer to a bowl and cover with the water. Place a plate on top of the chiles to keep them submerged in the water (if necessary, place something heavy, like a can or two, on top of the plate). Set aside for 30 minutes.

Drain off 2 cups of the water. Place the chiles and remaining water in a blender, along with the garlic, oil, tomato paste, cumin, oregano, and salt. Puree until smooth. Transfer the mixture to a 2- or 3-quart saucepan over high heat. Bring to a boil, reduce to a simmer, and cook 10 minutes.

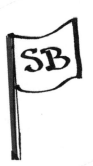

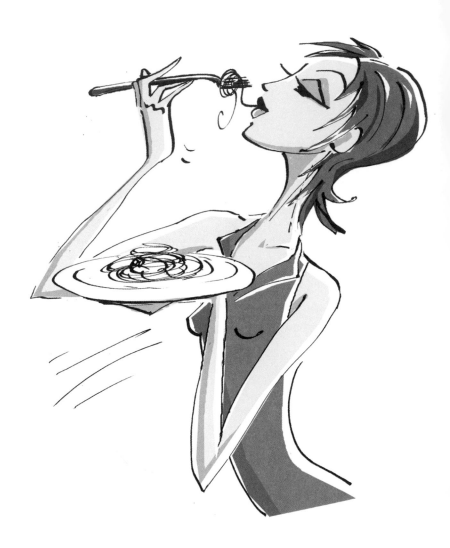

Italian
BITCH

Oh, Italian food, how we love thee.
When everyone was forsaking you for
"low carb" diets, we never turned our backs on you.
And we never will, Italian food. We never will.

East Coast Lasagna

Stuffed Shells

Penne with Butternut Squash,
Sage Pesto, and Almonds

Fettuccine Alfredo

Linguini with Pesto, Pine Nuts,
and Sun-dried Tomatoes

Eggplant Parmesan

East Coast Lasagna

Serves 8 to 12

6 quarts water

About 3 tablespoons fine sea salt

1 pound whole wheat or brown rice
lasagna noodles

5 cups Basic Red Sauce
(see page 156)

4 cups Tofu "Ricotta" (see page 158)

12 to 14 ounces vegan ground beef
(if frozen, no need to thaw)

10 ounces vegan mozzarella
cheese, shredded

Preheat oven to 350°F.

In an 8- to 10-quart stockpot over high heat, combine the water with about 3 tablespoons salt. Bring the water to a boil, add the lasagna noodles, and cook according to the package directions. When the pasta is done, drain it, briefly rinse it (just to make it cool enough to handle), and drain it again. Separate the noodles and lay them on foil, waxed paper, or parchment paper to keep them from sticking together.

Spread ½ cup of the Basic Red sauce in the bottom of a 13 x 9-inch pan. Top the sauce with some of the lasagna noodles, overlapping them slightly. Top the noodles with ⅓ of the Tofu Ricotta, ⅓ of the ground beef, and ⅓ of the cheese, spreading each layer of ingredients out evenly. Repeat the noodles, Tofu Ricotta, ground beef, and cheese layers two more times (you may not need all of the pasta).

Place the pan of lasagna on a rimmed baking sheet and bake until the tip of a knife inserted in the center of the lasagna comes out piping hot, 60 to 75 minutes. (Check on it periodically to make sure the cheese isn't burning. If it seems like it might, cover with foil until the final 15 minutes.) Remove the lasagna from the oven and let it sit 10 to 15 minutes before cutting and serving. Then chow the hell down!

Stuffed Shells with Red or White Sauce

Makes 22 to 24 shells,

to serve 6 to 8

3 quarts water

About 5 teaspoons fine sea salt

8 ounces whole wheat or brown rice
jumbo pasta shells

1 tablespoon refined coconut oil

½ onion, finely diced

2 cloves garlic, minced

2 cups Tofu "Ricotta"
(see page 158)

1 (10-ounce) package frozen
chopped spinach, thawed and
squeezed of excess water

2 tablespoons vegan Parmesan
cheese

2 tablespoons whole
wheat bread crumbs

¼ teaspoon pepper

2 cups Basic Red Sauce (see
page 156) or Savory White
Cream Sauce (see page 148)

Preheat oven to 350°F.

In a 4- to 6-quart stockpot over high heat, combine the water with about 1½ tablespoons of the salt. Bring the water to a boil, add the shells, and cook according to the package directions. When the pasta is done, drain it, briefly rinse it (just to make it cool enough to handle), and drain it again.

Meanwhile, heat the coconut oil in an 8- to 10-inch skillet over medium. Add the onions and cook, stirring occasionally, until tender, 4 to 6 minutes. Stir in the garlic and cook, stirring occasionally, 1 minute. Transfer the onion mixture to a large bowl and mix in the remaining ½ teaspoon salt, along with the Tofu Ricotta, spinach, cheese, bread crumbs, and pepper.

Spread about 1 cup of the Basic Red Sauce or Savory White Cream Sauce in the bottom of a 13 x 9-inch pan. Stuff each shell with about 2 tablespoons of the Tofu Ricotta mixture, arranging the stuffed shells on top of the sauce (you may not need all of the shells). Top each shell with a dollop of the remaining sauce, dividing it evenly. Cover the pan with foil and bake until the tip of a knife inserted in the center of one of the shells comes out piping hot, about 30 minutes.

Stuffed friggin' shells! Vegan style! Could you die or what?

Penne with Butternut Squash, Sage Pesto, and Almonds

Serves 4

3 quarts water

About 5 teaspoons fine sea salt

8 ounces whole wheat or
brown rice penne

2 tablespoons refined coconut oil

1½ pounds butternut squash,
peeled, seeded, and cut into
¼ inch thick sticks

2 shallots, thinly sliced

¼ teaspoon pepper

½ cup Sage Pesto (see page 155)

¼ cup sliced almonds,
toasted (optional)

In a 4- to 6-quart stockpot over high heat, combine the water with about 1½ tablespoons salt. Bring the water to a boil, add the penne, and cook according to the package directions.

Meanwhile, heat the coconut oil in a 10- to 12-inch skillet over medium-high heat. Add the squash and cook, stirring occasionally, for 4 minutes. Stir in the shallots, pepper, and the remaining ½ teaspoon salt and cook, stirring occasionally, until the squash and shallots are tender, 1 to 2 minutes. Remove from the heat and set aside.

When the pasta is done, drain it, reserving ½ cup of the pasta cooking water. Return the pasta to the pot and stir in the pesto and the squash mixture. If it seems too dry, add ¼ to ½ cup of the pasta water. Transfer the pasta to plates or a platter, and if desired, garnish with almonds. Serve immediately.

Fettuccini Alfredo

Serves 3 to 4

3 quarts water

About 4¾ teaspoons fine sea salt

8 ounces whole wheat or brown rice
   fettuccini

¼ cup refined coconut oil

½ cup vegan creamer

¼ cup vegan Parmesan cheese

¼ teaspoon pepper

2 cups fresh peas, cooked, or
   frozen peas, thawed (optional)

In a 4- to 6-quart stockpot over high heat, combine the water with about 1½ tablespoons salt. Bring the water to a boil, add the fettuccini, and cook according to the package directions.

Meanwhile, in a 1- to 2-quart saucepan over medium heat, melt the coconut oil. When it's almost melted, whisk in the creamer, increase the heat to medium high, and bring to a simmer. Whisk in the Parmesan, pepper, and the remaining ¼ teaspoon of salt. Cover and set aside.

When the pasta is done, drain it, reserving ½ cup of the pasta cooking water. Return the pasta to the pot and stir in the sauce (re-whisk if it separated) and peas, if using. If it seems too dry, add ¼ to ½ cup of the pasta water. Transfer the pasta to plates or a platter and serve.

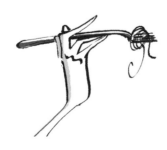

Linguini with Pesto, Pine Nuts, and Sun-dried Tomatoes

Serves 3 to 4

3 quarts water

About 1½ tablespoons fine sea salt

8 ounces whole wheat or
  brown rice linguini

½ cup Basil Pesto (see page 155)

½ cup oil-packed julienned
  sun-dried tomatoes, drained

½ cup pine nuts, toasted, divided

Zest of 1 lemon (optional)

¼ cup roughly chopped
  fresh basil leaves

In a 4- to 6-quart stockpot over high heat, combine the water with about 1½ tablespoons salt. Bring the water to a boil, add the linguini, and cook according to the package directions. When the pasta is done, drain it, reserving ½ cup of the pasta cooking water.

Return the pasta to the pot and stir in the pesto, sun-dried tomatoes, about ¾ of the pine nuts, and the lemon zest, if using. If the pasta seems too dry, add ¼ to ½ cup of the pasta water. Transfer the pasta to plates or a platter, garnish with the basil leaves and remaining pine nuts, and serve.

Eggplant Parmesan

> If you're one of those baby bitches— "I don't like eggplant" —now is the time to get over it.

**Serves 4 as an entree
or 8 as a side dish or appetizer**

¾ cup vegan Parmesan cheese

⅓ cup whole wheat bread crumbs

1 tablespoon granulated garlic powder

2 teaspoons fine sea salt

¾ teaspoon pepper

½ cup soy or rice milk

Refined coconut oil

1 eggplant (about 1½ pounds), cut
   crosswise into ½-inch slices

1½ cups Basic Red Sauce
   (see page 156)

¼ cup roughly chopped
   fresh basil leaves

4 ounces vegan mozzarella
   cheese, shredded

Preheat oven to 350°F.

In a shallow bowl, combine the Parmesan, bread crumbs, garlic powder, salt, and pepper. Place the soy or rice milk in another shallow bowl. Heat 3 to 4 tablespoons of oil, enough to coat the pan with a thin layer in a 10- or 12-inch nonstick skillet over medium.

One at a time, dip the eggplant slices in the soy or rice milk, then the bread-crumb mixture, pressing to thoroughly coat. Place the finished slices in the hot pan and cook about 3 minutes per side, or until browned on the outside and tender on the inside (you'll have to do more than one batch; wipe out the pan between batches and add more oil). Transfer the finished slices to a 2-quart casserole dish, arranging them into two layers. Top the eggplant with the sauce, spreading it evenly. Top the sauce with the basil and mozzarella, sprinkling both evenly. Bake until the sauce is hot and cheese is melted, about 20 minutes.

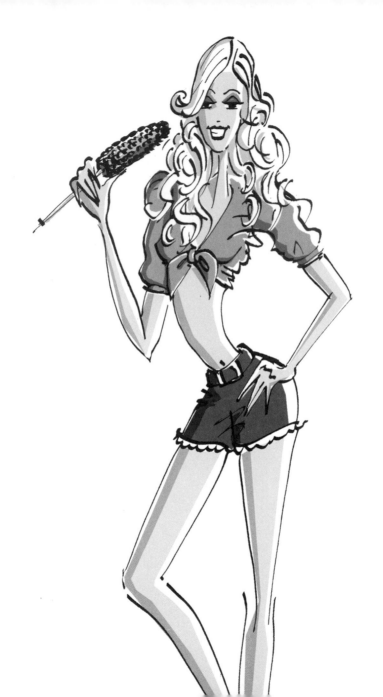

Down Home COOKIN'

If the shoe fits, wear it. And if you like to eat shit, eat it. And don't feel bad about it, neither. Here are a few old favorites that you might ordinarily feel guilty about eating. But now you can indulge without feeling fat or sick. (You can send us "thank-you" notes via www.SkinnyBitch.net.)

Macaroni and Four Cheeses

Oven-fried "Chicken" and Cornbread

Cha Cha Chili

Potatoes au Gratin

Shepherd's Pie

Cheezy Casserole

"Meatloaf" with Mashed Potatoes and Gravy

Sloppy Joes

Potato Skins with all the Fixin's

Macaroni and Four Cheeses

Serves 8

1 tablespoon refined coconut oil,
melted, or safflower oil, plus more
for the casserole dish
About 2 tablespoons fine sea salt
1 pound whole wheat or
brown rice elbow macaroni
2 (10-ounce) packages frozen
pureed winter squash
2 cups soy or rice milk
4 ounces vegan cheddar cheese,
shredded
2 ounces vegan Jack cheese,
shredded
4 ounces (about ½ cup)
vegan cream cheese
1½ teaspoons powdered mustard
⅛ teaspoon cayenne pepper
¼ cup whole wheat bread crumbs
2 tablespoons vegan Parmesan
cheese

Preheat oven to 375°F. Oil a 2-quart casserole dish; set aside.

In a 4- to 6-quart stockpot over high heat, combine 3 quarts of water with about 1½ tablespoons of the salt. Bring the water to a boil, add the macaroni, and cook according to the package directions.

Meanwhile, in a 3- to 4-quart saucepan over medium heat, combine the squash and milk, stirring and breaking up the squash with a spoon until the squash is defrosted. Increase the heat to medium-high and bring to a simmer, stirring occasionally. Remove from the heat and whisk in the cheddar, Jack, cream cheese, mustard, cayenne, and the remaining ½ tablespoon of salt.

When the pasta is done, drain it, then return the pasta to the pot. Stir the cheese sauce into the macaroni. Transfer the entire mixture to the prepared baking pan.

In a medium bowl, combine the bread crumbs, Parmesan, and the 1 tablespoon of oil. Sprinkle over the top of the macaroni and cheese. Place the casserole dish on a baking sheet and bake for 20 minutes, then broil for 2 to 3 minutes, or until the top is nicely browned.

If you don't experience multiple orgasms within the first three bites, you need to see your gyno.

Oven-fried "Chicken" and Cornbread

Serves 6 to 8

Refined coconut oil,
  for the baking sheet

¾ cup whole wheat panko
  (Japanese bread crumbs) or
  whole wheat bread crumbs

⅓ cup vegan chicken bouillon

3 tablespoons cornmeal

½ tablespoon fine sea salt

¾ teaspoon paprika

¼ teaspoon cayenne powder

1 cup soy milk

¾ cup brown rice flour

1½ pounds seitan (in larger blocks
  as opposed to thin slices), broken
  into large hunks

Cornbread (recipe follows)

Preheat oven to 450°F. Grease a large rimmed baking sheet with coconut oil; set aside.

In a shallow bowl, combine the panko, bouillon, corn meal, salt, paprika, and cayenne. Place the soy milk in a second bowl and the rice flour in a third. One at a time, dip the seitan pieces in the soy milk, the rice flour, the soy milk again, and then the panko mixture, pressing to thoroughly coat. Arrange the coated seitan on the prepared baking sheet and bake for 10 minutes. Turn the pieces over and cook another 10 minutes, or until slightly browned and heated throughout. Serve hot with cornbread.

CORNBREAD

Serves 6 to 8

1 tablespoon refined coconut oil,
   melted, or safflower oil, plus more
   for the baking pan
1½ cups yellow cornmeal
1¼ cups whole wheat pastry flour
¾ cup evaporated cane sugar
2 teaspoons baking powder
½ teaspoon fine sea salt
1½ cups soy milk
½ cup silken tofu

Preheat oven to 425°F. Oil a 13 x 9-inch baking pan; set aside.

In a large bowl, combine the cornmeal, flour, sugar, baking powder, and salt. In a blender, combine the milk, tofu, and the 1 tablespoon of the oil, pureeing until smooth. Add the milk mixture to the cornmeal mixture, stirring just until combined. Pour the batter into the prepared baking pan.

Bake the cornbread until golden brown—about 20 minutes. (It'll also begin to pull away from the edges of the pan and spring back when lightly pressed in the center.) Transfer to a cooling rack for 10 minutes, then remove the cornbread from the pan and return to rack to cool completely.

The cornbread can be made in advance and kept at room temperature overnight or in the freezer for up to 1 month.

Cha Cha Chile

Toot, toot, baby. Toot, toot.

Serves 6 to 8

2 cups dry red kidney beans

1 tablespoon refined coconut oil

2 onions, cut into ¼-inch dice

2 cloves garlic, minced

¼ cup chili powder

½ tablespoon fine sea salt

1 teaspoon pepper

1 teaspoon dried oregano

½ teaspoon dried sage

½ teaspoon ground cumin

Pinch cayenne pepper

1 (14½-ounce) can chopped
    tomatoes

½ cup medium-grain brown rice

1 red, green, or yellow bell pepper,
    cut into ¼-inch dice

1 carrot, shredded

Chopped red onion,
    for serving (optional)

Shredded vegan cheddar cheese,
    for serving (optional)

Vegan sour cream, for serving (optional)

In a 4- to 6-quart stockpot, combine the beans and enough cold water to cover by 2 inches. Cover and refrigerate for at least 8 hours or overnight. (Alternately, bring to a boil over high heat, cover, remove from heat, and let sit for 1 hour.)

Drain the beans, return them to the stockpot, and cover with water by 1 inch. Place the pot over high heat, bring to a boil, and reduce to a simmer.

Meanwhile, in an 8- to 10-inch skillet over medium, heat the oil. Add the onions and cook, stirring occasionally, for 4 minutes. Add the garlic, chili powder, salt, pepper, oregano, sage, cumin, and cayenne and cook for 1 minute. Add the onion mixture to the beans, along with the tomatoes and rice. Cook for 30 minutes.

Add the bell pepper and cook for 15 minutes. Add the carrot and cook about 5 minutes, until the beans and rice are tender.

Serve with red onions, shredded cheese, and sour cream, if desired.

Potatoes au Gratin

Serves 8 to 10

4 medium russet potatoes
(about 3 pounds), sliced very thin

1 teaspoon fine sea salt

½ teaspoon pepper

4 ounces vegan cheddar cheese,
shredded

2½ to 3 cups soy creamer

2 tablespoons arrowroot or
7 teaspoons cornstarch

1½ cups cornflake cereal

Preheat oven to 375°F.

In a 2-quart casserole dish, evenly layer half of the potatoes in a scallop pattern. (You may have to make a couple of layers.) Sprinkle the potatoes with half of the salt, half of the pepper, and half of the cheese. Add the remaining potatoes, evenly layering them in a scallop pattern.

Combine 2½ cups of the creamer with the arrowroot or cornstarch, whisking to dissolve the arrowroot. Pour the mixture over the potatoes. Use a spatula to press the potatoes down into the cream; they should be just barely submerged. If not, add more cream. Sprinkle with the remaining salt, the remaining pepper, and the remaining cheese. Cover and bake for 45 minutes.

Meanwhile, crush the cornflakes, by hand or by pulsing in a food processor, to very coarse crumbs.

Remove the casserole from the oven and use a spatula to moisten the top layer of potatoes by pressing them into the cream. Sprinkle on the cornflakes and bake, uncovered, another 30 to 45 minutes, until the liquid has become a thick sauce, the potatoes are tender, and the cornflakes are browned. Serve warm.

Shepherd's Pie

Serves 6 to 8

1 tablespoon refined coconut oil

2 shallots, thinly sliced

2 cloves garlic, minced

1 teaspoon herbes de Provence
(see page 62)

1 teaspoon fine sea salt

1½ cups lentils

About 3 cups low-sodium
vegetable stock

2 tomatoes, cut into ½-inch dice

1 bunch (about ½ pound) chard,
leafy parts only, cut into ½-inch
strips

6 cups Mashed Potatoes
(see page 119)

Preheat oven to 350°F.

Heat the oil in a 4- to 6-quart stockpot over medium. Add the shallots and cook, stirring occasionally, for 1 minute. Add the garlic, herbes de Provence, and ½ teaspoon of the salt and cook, stirring occasionally, for 1 minute, or until the shallots are browned. Add the lentils and 2½ cups of the vegetable stock, increase the heat to high, and bring to a boil. Reduce to a simmer, cover, and cook until the lentils are tender and the stock is absorbed, 35 to 40 minutes. Stir in the tomatoes and transfer the lentil mixture to a 2-quart casserole dish, spreading it evenly.

Add the remaining ½ cup of stock to the pot and return it to high heat. When the stock comes to a boil, add the chard and the remaining ½ teaspoon of salt. Cook, stirring occasionally, until the chard is tender and the liquid has been absorbed, about 4 minutes. (If the pan gets dry before the chard is cooked, add more stock, 2 tablespoons at a time.) Add the chard to the casserole dish, spreading it evenly. Top with the mashed potatoes, spreading them evenly.

Place the casserole dish on a rimmed baking sheet and bake until thoroughly heated through and the potatoes are slightly browned, about 30 minutes. Serve warm.

If you're feeling fancy, instead of a 2-quart casserole dish, you can serve this in eight 1-cup ramekins. Divide the ingredients among them and check them after only 20 minutes in the oven.

Cheezy Casserole

Serves 6 to 8

Refined coconut oil,
   for the casserole dish

1½ cups short grain brown rice

3 quarts plus 3 cups water

About 4¾ teaspoons fine sea salt

8 ounces (or four to six) red
   potatoes, cut into ¾-inch cubes

2 carrots, cut on a diagonal
   into ¼-inch slices

½ red onion, cut into ¾-inch dice

4 ounces sugar snap peas, cut
   crosswise in half

1 broccoli crown, cut into bite-sized
   florets (about 2½ cups)

14 to 16 ounces firm, extra firm, or
   baked tofu, cut into ½-inch cubes

2¾ cups Cheezy Sauce
   (see page 150)

¼ cup coarsely chopped
   Italian parsley

⅓ cup sliced almonds

Tamari or soy sauce,
   for serving (optional)

Preheat oven to 375°F. Grease a 2-quart casserole dish. Line a large bowl with one or two paper towels.

In a 2-quart saucepan over high heat, combine the rice, 3 cups of the water, and ¼ teaspoon of the salt. Bring to a boil, reduce the heat to a simmer, cover, and cook until the water is absorbed and the rice is tender, about 45 minutes. Remove from the heat and let the rice stand, covered, at least 10 minutes.

Meanwhile, in a 4- to 6-quart stockpot over high heat, combine the remaining 3 quarts of water with about 1½ table-spoons salt. Bring the water to a boil. Add the potatoes and cook until they are soft but still holding their shape, about 5 minutes. Use a slotted spoon or hand-held strainer to remove the potatoes to the prepared bowl. Then remove the paper towels. Add the carrots and onion to the stockpot and cook until tender, about 2 minutes. Use the same slotted spoon to remove the carrots and onions, adding them to the bowl. Add the snap peas and broccoli to the stockpot and cook until tender, about 1 minute. Remove the snap peas and broccoli, adding them to the bowl.

Add the cooked rice, tofu, Cheezy Sauce, and parsley to the vegetables, tossing until combined. Transfer the mixture to the prepared casserole dish. Place the casserole on a rimmed baking sheet and bake for 30 minutes. Sprinkle almonds on top and bake for 15 minutes, or until the almonds are toasted and the tip of a knife inserted into the center of the casserole comes out piping hot. If using, pass the tamari or soy sauce at the table.

"Meatloaf"
with Mashed Potatoes and Gravy

Serves 6

1 tablespoon refined coconut oil,
   plus more for the pan
1 carrot, cut into ¼-inch dice
1 celery stalk, cut into ¼-inch dice
1 onion, cut into ¼-inch dice
3 ounces cremini, shiitake, or
   portobello mushrooms, cut into
   ¼-inch dice (about 2 cups)
2 cloves garlic, minced
2 teaspoons fine sea salt
1 teaspoon pepper
2 slices vegan whole wheat bread
1 cup toasted walnuts
2 (14-ounce) packages Gimme
   Lean vegan ground beef
½ cup rolled oats
½ cup ketchup
2 tablespoons chopped
   fresh Italian parsley
6 cups Mashed Potatoes
   (recipe follows)
2½ cups Brown Gravy (see page 149)

Preheat oven to 375°F. Oil a 10 x 4 x 3 inch loaf pan.

In an 8- to 10-inch skillet over medium heat, melt the oil. Add the carrot and celery and cook, stirring occasionally, for 2 minutes. Add the onion and cook, stirring occasionally, for 3 minutes. Add the mushrooms, garlic, salt, and pepper and cook, stirring occasionally, until the vegetables are crisp-tender and any liquid the mushrooms have released is cooked off, about 2 minutes. Remove from heat and allow to cool slightly.

Meanwhile, in a food processor, combine the bread and walnuts, pulsing to form a coarse meal. Transfer the mixture to a large bowl and add the beef, oats, ketchup, parsley, and the vegetable mixture. Use your hands to mix well. Transfer the loaf mixture to the prepared pan, spread it into an even layer, and bake for 45 minutes, until the tip of a knife inserted into the center comes out piping hot.

Let the loaf sit 5 minutes before turning it out onto a serving plate. Cut into slices and serve with Mashed Potatoes and Brown Gravy. If you're not drooling, check your pulse.

....

MASHED POTATOES

Makes 6 cups, serves 6 to 8

2 quarts water

About 3½ teaspoons fine sea salt

3 large russet potatoes (about 2¼ pounds), cut into 1½-inch cubes

1 cup soy or rice milk

3 tablespoons vegan butter

½ teaspoon pepper

In a 4- to 6-quart stockpot, combine the water and about 1 tablespoon of the salt. Add the potatoes and place the pot over high heat. Bring to a boil, reduce to a simmer, and cook until the potatoes are very tender, 15 to 20 minutes.

Drain the potatoes and return them to the pot. Add the milk, the remaining ½ teaspoon salt, the butter, and pepper. Then mash, bitches, mash!

Sloppy Joes

Serves 4 to 6

2 tablespoons refined coconut oil

1 green bell pepper, cut into
⅟₄-inch dice

1 stalk celery, halved lengthwise
and cut into ⅟₄-inch slices

2 large onions, cut into ⅟₄-inch dice

4 ounces thinly sliced white or
cremini (brown) mushrooms
(about 2 cups)

1 teaspoon chili powder

½ teaspoon fine sea salt

¼ teaspoon pepper

2 cups water

1 (15-ounce) can tomato sauce

¼ cup Bragg's Liquid Aminos (or 8
teaspoons tamari or soy sauce)

¼ cup ketchup

1½ cups textured soy protein

4 to 6 vegan whole wheat
hamburger buns

2 to 3 tablespoons vegan Parmesan
cheese, for serving (optional)

Heat the coconut oil in a 10- to 12-inch skillet over medium high. Add the bell pepper and celery and cook, stirring occasionally, for 2 minutes. Add the onion and cook, stirring occasionally, for 4 minutes. Add the mushroom, chili powder, salt, and pepper and cook, stirring occasionally, for 2 minutes. Stir in the water, tomato sauce, Bragg's Liquid Aminos or tamari or soy sauce, and ketchup. Stir in the textured soy protein, increase the heat to high, and bring to a boil. Reduce to a simmer and cook, stirring occasionally, for 20 minutes.

Meanwhile, split and toast the buns.

To serve, place two bun halves on each plate, open faced. Top the buns with the Sloppy Joe mixture, dividing evenly. Sprinkle with Parmesan cheese, if using, and serve.

Serve with potato salad (see page 66) and dill pickle chips.

Potato Skins with all the Fixin's

Serves 4 to 6 as an appetizer

3 medium russet potatoes,
  scrubbed and patted dry

Refined coconut oil, for the potatoes
  and the baking sheet

6 slices vegan bacon, cooked
  according to package directions

4 ounces shredded vegan cheddar
  cheese (about 1¼ cups)

4 ounces shredded vegan Jack
  cheese (about 1¼ cups)

1 tablespoon chopped fresh parsley

½ teaspoon fine sea salt

¼ teaspoon pepper

3 scallions, thinly sliced

¾ cup vegan sour cream

Preheat oven to 425 °F.

Rub the potatoes with oil and place them on a large rimmed baking sheet. Bake until the potatoes are tender, about 1 hour. Set the potatoes aside until they're cool enough to handle, but keep the oven on.

Meanwhile, chop the bacon. In a medium bowl, combine the bacon, cheddar cheese, Jack cheese, and parsley; set aside.

Cut each potato lengthwise into quarters. Scoop out the insides, leaving a ¼-inch layer of potato on the skins (save the insides for another use). Oil the baking sheet. Place the skins, skin side down and one inch apart, on the sheet. Sprinkle with the salt, pepper, and the cheese mixture, dividing them evenly. Bake until the skins are crisp and the cheese is melted, about 15 minutes.

Transfer the skins to plates or a platter. Sprinkle with the scallions and dollop with sour cream, dividing evenly.

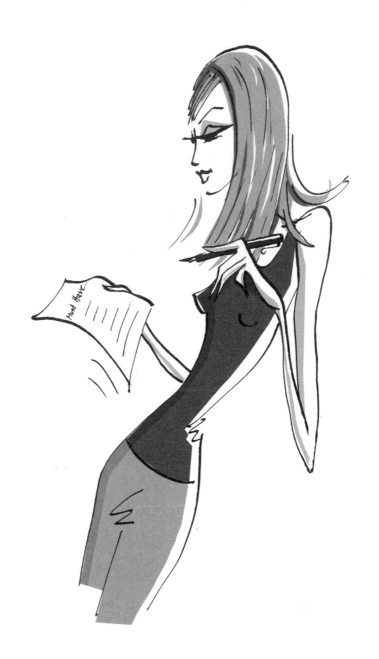

Skinny Bitch
STAPLE MEALS

*These hearty, wholesome, satisfying meals
are the staples to get you through day-to-day life.*

Steamed Veggies and Tofu with Brown Rice

Double-dip Fondue

Roasted Sausage, Peppers, Onions,
and Garlic over Soft Polenta

Big-ass Veggie Burrito

Smoked Tofu Stir-Fry

Summer Garden Pasta

Waldorf Wheat Berry Salad

French Lentil Salad

Tamari-roasted Root Vegetables with Cashew Millet

Balsamic Portobello Mushrooms
over Grilled Vegetable Couscous

Spaghetti Squash with Spicy Braised
Greens, Raisins, and Pine Nuts

Hummus, Tempeh, and Cucumber Wrap

Green Goddess Pasta

Chicken Square Meal with White Beans,
Quinoa Pilaf, and Asparagus

Steamed Veggies and Tofu with Brown Rice

Serves 4 to 6

1½ cups medium grain brown rice

3½ cups water, plus more for steaming

¼ teaspoon fine sea salt

½ cup tahini (sesame seed paste)

¼ cup sesame oil

6 tablespoons Bragg's Liquid
Aminos, plus more for the table (or
4 tablespoons tamari or soy sauce)

2 carrots, cut into ¼-inch slices

¼ head cauliflower, cut into bite-
sized florets (about 2 cups)

¼ head red cabbage (about 6
ounces), cut into ¼-inch strips

¼ bunch kale (about 4 ounces or four
to six leaves) cut into ½-inch strips

1 broccoli crown, cut into bite-sized
florets (about 2½ cups)

7 to 8 ounces firm or extra firm tofu,
cut into ¼-inch slices, then cut on
a diagonal into triangles

¼ cup raw pine nuts

In a 2-quart saucepan over high heat, combine the rice, 3 cups of the water, and the salt. Bring to a boil, reduce the heat to a simmer, cover, and cook until the water is absorbed and the rice is tender, about 45 minutes. Remove from the heat and let the rice stand, covered, at least 10 minutes.

Meanwhile, in a small bowl, whisk together the tahini, sesame oil, ¼ cup of the Bragg's Liquid Aminos (or 8 teaspoons of tamari or soy sauce), and the remaining ½ cup of water; set aside.

In a pot fitted with a steamer insert, bring 1 inch of water and the remaining 2 tablespoons of Bragg's Liquid Aminos (or 4 teaspoons of the tamari or soy sauce) to a boil. Arrange the carrot and cauliflower in the insert and steam for 3 minutes. Add the cabbage, kale, broccoli, and tofu and steam for 3 minutes, until the vegetables are tender and the tofu is heated through.

To serve, place the rice on plates or a platter and top with the vegetable mixture, tahini sauce, and pine nuts. Pass any remaining sauce and additional Bragg's Liquid Aminos at the table.

Uhhh!!! This dish tastes so simple, pure, and good it makes us mad!

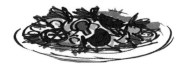

Double-dip Fondue

Serves 6

2 cups bite-sized broccoli
  florets, blanched

2 cups bite-sized cauliflower
  florets, blanched

2 red bell peppers,
  cut into 1-inch dice

12 bite-sized potatoes, cooked

1½ cups dry white wine

1 tablespoon coarse nutritional yeast

1 clove garlic, pressed or finely
  minced

2 teaspoons Bragg's Liquid
  Aminos, (or 1¼ teaspoons tamari
  or soy sauce)

6 teaspoons arrowroot or
  7 teaspoons cornstarch

6 teaspoons water, divided

1 pound vegan Jack cheese, shredded

2½ cups low-sodium vegetable stock

2 (14- to 16-ounce packages)
  firm or extra firm tofu, pressed
  and cut into ¾-inch cubes

To blanch vegetables: Bring a pot of well-salted water (about ½ tablespoon fine sea salt per quart of water) to a boil. Add the vegetables and cook until crisp-tender, 1 to 3 minutes depending on the vegetable and the size (blanch different vegetables separately since cooking times may vary). Remove with a slotted spoon (if blanching other vegetables) or drain.

To make the cheese fondue: In a 3- to 4-quart saucepan over medium heat, combine the wine, nutritional yeast, garlic, and ½ teaspoon of the Bragg's Liquid Aminos (or ¼ teaspoon tamari or soy sauce), and bring to a simmer.

Meanwhile, in a small bowl, whisk together 4 teaspoons of the arrowroot, (or 4½ teaspoons of the cornstarch)and 4 teaspoons of the water.

About a cup at a time, add the cheese to the saucepan, whisking until all the cheese is incorporated and the mixture is smooth. Whisk in the arrowroot mixture. Bring to a simmer and cook, whisking occasionally, until thickened, 5 to 8 minutes. Transfer to a fondue pot set over a flame.

To make the broth fondue: In a 3- to 4-quart saucepan over medium high heat, combine the stock and the remaining 1½ teaspoons Bragg's Liquid Aminos (or 1 teaspoon tamari or soy sauce), and bring to a simmer.

Meanwhile, in a small bowl, whisk together the remaining 2 teaspoons arrowroot (or 2½ teaspoons of the cornstarch) and the remaining 2 teaspoons water. Whisk the arrowroot mixture into the stock mixture, stirring until slightly thickened. Transfer to a fondue pot set over a flame.

Arrange the broccoli, cauliflower, bell pepper, potatoes, and tofu on plates or a platter and serve.

FYI: The broth is more like a flavorful liquid to warm the veggies and tofu in, while the cheese is more of a dipping thing.

Other things that'd be good to dip: cubed apples, pears, bread, etc.

Roasted Sausage, Peppers, Onions, and Garlic over Soft Polenta

Serves 4

12 cloves garlic

4 red, yellow, or green bell peppers, or a combination, cut into ¾-inch strips

2 onions, quartered and cut into ¾-inch strips

2 tablespoons refined coconut oil, melted, or safflower oil

1 teaspoon fine sea salt

¼ teaspoon pepper

4 (12 to 16 ounces total) vegan Italian sausages, cut diagonally into ¾-inch slices

4 to 4½ cups low-sodium vegetable stock

1 cup polenta

⅔ cup vegan Parmesan cheese

Aged balsamic vinegar or extra virgin olive oil, for drizzling (optional)

Preheat oven to 425° F.

In a large bowl, combine the garlic, bell peppers, onions, oil, ½ teaspoon of the salt, and the pepper, tossing to coat. Transfer the mixture to a rimmed baking sheet and cook for 20 minutes, until the garlic and vegetables are tender.

Stir in the sausages and cook until the vegetables and sausages start to brown, 15 to 20 minutes.

Meanwhile, in a 2- to 3-quart saucepan over medium-high heat, combine 4 cups of the stock and the remaining ½ teaspoon of salt and bring to a boil. Add the polenta in a thin stream, stirring constantly. Return to a boil, reduce to a simmer, cover, and cook until the polenta is tender, 8 to 10 minutes. If the polenta seems too thick, add more stock, ¼ cup at a time. Remove the saucepan from the heat and stir in ⅓ cup of the Parmesan.

To serve, transfer the polenta to 4 serving bowls and top with the sausage and vegetable mixture, dividing evenly. Pass the remaining ⅓ cup of Parmesan and balsamic vinegar or olive oil, if using, at the table.

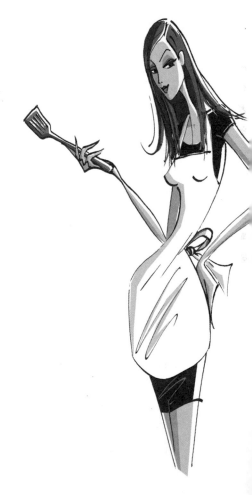

Big-Ass Veggie Burrito

Makes 4

1 cup brown rice

2 cups water

½ teaspoon plus a pinch fine sea salt

1 (15-ounce) can black beans

1 tablespoon refined coconut oil

1 yellow squash, cut into
  ½-inch cubes

1 green bell pepper, cut into
  ½-inch dice

1 mild green chile, such as pasilla or
  Anaheim, cut into ½-inch dice

½ red onion, cut into ½-inch dice

1 zucchini, quartered lengthwise
  and cut into ½-inch slices

4 cloves garlic, minced

1 teaspoon chili powder

1 teaspoon ground coriander

1 teaspoon ground cumin

2 tomatoes, cut into ½-inch cubes

2 tablespoons lime juice

4 (12- to 14-inch) whole wheat
  tortillas, heated

1 pound vegan cheddar or Jack
  cheese, shredded

½ cup coarsely chopped fresh
  cilantro

2 scallions, thinly sliced

In a 1- to 2-quart saucepan over high heat, combine the rice, water, and a pinch of the salt. Bring to a boil, reduce the heat to a simmer, cover, and cook until the water is absorbed and the rice is tender, about 45 minutes. Remove from the heat and let the rice stand, covered, at least 10 minutes.

Meanwhile, place the beans and their liquid in a 1-quart saucepan over medium heat. Bring to a simmer, reduce the heat to low, and cook until the beans are heated through, about 3 minutes. Cover and set aside.

Heat the coconut oil in a 10- to 12-inch skillet over medium high. Add the squash and cook, stirring occasionally, for 1 minute. Add the bell pepper and chile and cook, stirring occasionally for 1 minute. Add the onion and cook, stirring occasionally, for 2 minutes. Add the zucchini, garlic, chili powder, coriander, cumin, and the remaining ½ teaspoon of salt and cook, stirring occasionally, for 4 minutes, or until all the vegetables are crisp tender. Stir in the tomatoes. Reduce the heat to low, cover, and cook for 4 minutes, until the vegetables are very soft. Stir in the lime juice.

To serve, lay a tortilla on a work surface and top with ¼ of the rice, arranging it in a column down the middle of the tortilla, 2 inches from either edge. Top with ¼ of the beans, ¼ of the vegetable mixture, ¼ of the cheese, ¼ of the cilantro, and ¼ of the scallions. Fold one side of the tortilla up and over the fillings, fold in the edges, and continue rolling the tortilla to the other side, making a tight bundle. Transfer the burrito to a plate, seam down. Repeat with remaining tortillas.

Beans, onions, garlic. You may want to stay in for the night after this one.

Smoked Tofu Stir-fry

Serves 3 to 4

1 cup brown basmati rice

1¾ cups water

Pinch fine sea salt

⅔ cup vegetable stock

¼ cup mirin (see note on page 89)

2 tablespoons tamari or soy sauce, plus more for the table

1 tablespoon arrowroot or 3½ teaspoons cornstarch

1 tablespoon refined coconut oil

½ white or yellow onion, halved and cut into ¼-inch slices

2 heads baby bok choy (about 12 ounces), halved lengthwise then cut crosswise into ½-inch slices

2 cloves garlic, thinly sliced

1 tablespoon minced ginger

1 portobello mushroom, halved and cut into ¼-inch slices

8 shiitake mushrooms, stemmed and thinly sliced

8 white or cremini (brown) mushrooms, thinly sliced

1 (6- to 8-ounce package) smoked tofu, cut into bite-sized ¼-inch slices

3 scallions, cut into 2-inch lengths, white parts halved lengthwise

In a 1- to 2-quart saucepan over high heat, combine the rice, water, and salt. Bring to a boil, reduce the heat to a simmer, cover, and cook until the water is absorbed and the rice is tender, about 30 minutes. Remove from the heat and let the rice stand, covered, at least 10 minutes.

Meanwhile, in a small bowl, whisk together the stock, mirin, tamari or soy sauce, and arrowroot or cornstarch; set aside.

Heat the coconut oil in a 12- to 14-inch wok or skillet over high. Add the onion and stir-fry for 1 minute. Add the bok choy, garlic, and ginger and stir-fry for 1 minute. Add the portobello and stir fry for 1 minute. Add the remaining mushrooms and stir-fry for 3 minutes, or until all the mushrooms are tender. Stir in the stock mixture and the tofu and stir-fry until the tofu is heated through and the sauce has thickened, 1 to 2 minutes. Stir in the scallions.

To serve, arrange the rice on plates or a platter and top with the mushroom mixture. Pass additional tamari or soy sauce at the table.

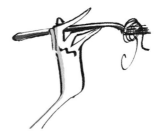

Summer Garden Pasta

Serves 4

3 quarts water

About 5 teaspoons fine sea salt

8 ounces whole wheat or brown rice
linguini or fettuccini

¼ cup refined coconut oil

6 shallots, thinly sliced

1 zucchini, halved lengthwise
and thinly sliced

1 yellow squash, halved lengthwise
and thinly sliced

4 cloves garlic, thinly sliced

¼ teaspoon pepper

2 pounds tomatoes — red, yellow,
or a combination — seeded
and cut into coarse ¼-inch dice
(about three cups)

½ cup thinly sliced fresh basil leaves

2 tablespoons chopped fresh
oregano

¼ cup extra virgin olive oil

1 to 2 tablespoons vegan Parmesan
(optional)

In a 4- to 6-quart stockpot over high heat, combine the water with about 1½ tablespoons of the salt. Bring the water to a boil, add the pasta, and cook according to the package directions.

Meanwhile, heat the coconut oil in a 10- to 12-inch skillet over medium high heat. Add the shallots and cook, stirring occasionally, for 3 minutes. Add the zucchini, squash, garlic, pepper, and the remaining ½ teaspoon salt and cook, stirring occasionally, until the vegetables are tender, about 2 minutes. Reduce the heat to medium and add the tomatoes, basil, and oregano, stirring until the tomatoes are heated through, about 2 minutes.

When the pasta is done, drain it. Transfer the pasta to plates or a platter and top with the tomato mixture. Drizzle with olive oil, sprinkle with Parmesan, if using, and serve.

Waldorf Wheat Berry Salad

Serves 6 to 8

1 cup hard wheat berries (see note)

3 cups water, plus more for soaking

⅓ cup safflower oil

¼ cup apple juice

2 tablespoons rice vinegar

2 tablespoons agave nectar

¾ teaspoon fine sea salt

½ teaspoon pepper

2 celery stalks, thinly sliced

2 scallions, thinly sliced

1 sweet-tart apple, such as Fuji,
   Jonathan, or McIntosh,
   cut into ½-inch cubes

½ small red onion,
   cut into ¼-inch dice

½ cup dried cranberries

½ cup chopped pecans

½ cup chopped fresh Italian parsley

HARD WHEAT BERRIES
are available in the bulk section
of natural food stores and
many supermarkets.

In a 2- to 3-quart saucepan, combine the wheat berries and enough water to cover by 2 inches and soak, refrigerated, for 6 hours or overnight. (If you don't have time for the overnight drama, use ½ cup more water and cook for thirty minutes more, or until tender.)

Drain the wheat berries, return them to the pot, and add the 3 cups of water. Bring to a boil over high heat, reduce the heat to a simmer, cover, and cook for 50 to 60 minutes, until the berries are tender.

Meanwhile, in a small bowl, whisk together the safflower oil, apple juice, rice vinegar, agave, salt, and pepper. Once the berries are cooked, drain any water left in the pot and transfer the berries to a large bowl. Toss with about half the dressing and set aside to cool to room temperature.

Once the berries are cool, stir in the ingredients and remaining dressing, tossing gently. Serve cold.

French Lentil Salad

Serves 6 to 8

1 cup French green lentils (see note)

2 cups water

6 tablespoons extra virgin olive oil

2 tablespoons white wine vinegar
or champagne vinegar

½ tablespoon fresh chopped or
½ teaspoon dry tarragon

1 teaspoon Dijon mustard

1 teaspoon fine sea salt

½ teaspoon pepper

2 tomatoes, cut into ½-inch dice

2 large Belgian endive (about 8
ounces), halved lengthwise and
cut into ½-inch slices

1 green bell pepper,
cut into ½-inch dice

1 yellow bell pepper, cut into
½-inch dice

½ cup chopped fresh Italian parsley

In a 1- to 2-quart saucepan over high, combine the lentils and water and bring to a boil. Reduce the heat to a simmer, cover, and cook 35 to 45 minutes, until the lentils are al dente, tender but not mushy.

Meanwhile, in a small bowl, whisk together the olive oil, vinegar, tarragon, mustard, salt, and pepper.

Once the lentils are cooked, drain any water left in the pot and transfer the lentils to a large bowl. Toss with about half the dressing and set aside to cool to room temperature.

Once the lentils are cool, stir in the tomatoes, endive, bell peppers, and parsley. Add the remaining dressing, tossing gently. Serve cold or at room temperature.

Don't get all psycho if you can't find French green lentils. This can be made with brown, pink, or regular green lentils, as well.

Tamari-roasted Root Vegetables with Cashew Millet

Serves 6

4 beets (about 24 ounces), trimmed,
 peeled, and cut into ¾-inch cubes
4 rutabagas (about 24 ounces),
 trimmed, peeled, and cut into
 ¾-inch cubes
4 turnips (about 24 ounces),
 trimmed, peeled, and cut into
 ¾-inch cubes
3 tablespoons tamari,
 plus more for the table
1 tablespoon safflower oil
3¾ cups low-sodium
 vegetable stock
1½ cups hulled millet
¼ teaspoon fine sea salt
½ cup chopped cashews

Preheat oven to 375°F.

In a large bowl, combine the beets, rutabagas, turnips, tamari, and safflower oil. Spread the mixture onto two large rimmed baking sheets and bake for 30 minutes. One pan at a time, remove the pans from the oven, toss the vegetables, and spread them back out. Cook for another 30 minutes, or until the vegetables are tender and nicely caramelized.

Meanwhile, in a 3- to 4-quart saucepan over high heat, combine the stock, millet, and salt. Bring to a boil, reduce the heat to a simmer, cover, and cook for 15 minutes, or until the millet is tender. Remove from the heat, fluff with a fork, cover, and set aside until the vegetables are done.

To serve, transfer the millet to plates or a platter, top with the vegetables, and sprinkle with cashews. Pass additional tamari at the table.

Balsamic Portobello Mushrooms over Grilled Vegetable Couscous

Serves 4

¾ cup coconut oil, melted,
  or safflower oil

½ cup balsamic vinegar

2 tablespoons maple syrup

2 tablespoons chopped
  fresh rosemary

½ teaspoon freshly ground
  black pepper

2¼ teaspoons fine sea salt

1 small red onion

4 portobello mushrooms

1 medium zucchini, cut lengthwise
  into ½-inch slices

1 yellow squash, cut lengthwise
  into ½-inch slices

1¼ cups water

1 cup couscous

In a medium bowl, whisk together the oil, balsamic vinegar, maple syrup, rosemary, pepper, and ½ tablespoon of the salt; set aside.

Trim the stem end off of onion and peel. Cut the onion into 8 wedges, each with a bit of the root end holding it together. Place the onion, portobellos, zucchini, and squash in a large, resealable bag and add the balsamic mixture. Press the air out of the bag, seal, and set aside for 2 to 4 hours, turning occasionally.

Prepare an outdoor or stovetop grill to medium heat (it's at the right temperature when you can hold your hand grate-level for 4 seconds).

Remove the vegetables from the bag and reserve 2 tablespoons of the marinade (save the rest for another use). Grill the vegetables for 8 to 10 minutes, turning once, until well-marked and tender.

(If you don't have a grill, use two to three skillets with a little oil in the bottom over medium-high heat. Just be sure not to crowd the veggies in there or they'll steam instead of sear.

Meanwhile, in a 2- to 3-quart saucepan over medium heat, bring the water and the remaining ¾ teaspoon of salt to a boil. Stir in the couscous, cover, remove from the heat, and let stand for 5 minutes.

Once the vegetables have cooked, coarsely chop the onion, zucchini, and squash. Stir the chopped vegetables into the couscous, along with the reserved marinade. Cut the portobellos into thick slices.

Arrange the couscous on plates or a platter, top with the portobellos and any accumulated juices, and serve.

Spaghetti Squash with Spicy Braised Greens, Raisins, and Pine Nuts

Serves 4

½ of a 4-pound spaghetti squash, with the seeds scraped out (see note)

Water for the baking pan

2 tablespoons refined coconut oil

2 cloves garlic, minced

1 to 2 canned chipotle chiles in adobo sauce, seeded and minced

1½ bunches (about 12 ounces) kale, chard, mustard greens, collard greens, or a combination, cut into ½-inch strips

1 to 1½ cups low-sodium vegetable stock

¾ teaspoon fine sea salt

⅓ cup raisins

¼ cup pine nuts

2 tablespoons extra virgin olive oil

Preheat oven to 375°F.

Place the squash flesh down in a 13 x 9-inch baking pan. Add ¼ inch of water and bake until the squash is easily pierced with a fork, 50 to 60 minutes.

Meanwhile, heat the coconut oil in a 4- to 6-quart stockpot over medium. Add the garlic and chipotle and cook for 1 minute. Add the greens, handfuls at a time, stirring until they're all in the pot. Add 1 cup of the stock, ½ teaspoon of the salt, and the raisins. Increase the heat to high and bring to a boil. Reduce the heat to a simmer, cover, and cook until the greens are tender, about 10 minutes, or 15 to 20 minutes for collard greens. (If the pan gets dry before the chard is cooked, add more stock, 2 tablespoons at a time.) Stir in 3 tablespoons of the pine nuts.

When the squash is done, use a fork to separate the strands into a large bowl.

Add the olive oil and the remaining ¼ teaspoon of salt and toss gently.

Transfer the "spaghetti" to plates or a platter, top with the greens mixture, garnish with the remaining 1 tablespoon of pine nuts, and serve.

We're not dumb broads. We know that "½ of a 4-pound squash" means you could just buy a 2-pound squash. But a larger squash merits longer, thicker strands of spaghetti than a whole small squash. So do what you're told— just save the other half for another use

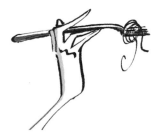

Hummus, Tempeh, and Cucumber Wrap

Makes 4

1 tablespoon refined coconut oil

½ teaspoon garlic powder

¼ teaspoon ground coriander

2 tablespoons tamari or soy sauce

1 (8-ounce) package tempeh, cut
lengthwise into ¼-inch strips

4 (9- to 10-inch) whole wheat tortillas

1 cup hummus

1 cucumber, peeled and cut
diagonally into ¼-inch slices

1 romaine heart, cut into ½-inch strips

¼ cup bottled vinaigrette dressing,
whatever kind you like

Heat the coconut oil in a 10- to 12-inch skillet over medium heat. Stir in the garlic powder, coriander, and tamari or soy sauce. Add the tempeh and cook 1½ to 2 minutes per side, until browned.

To serve, lay a tortilla on a work surface and spread it with ¼ of the hummus. Arrange ¼ of the tempeh in a column down the middle of the tortilla, leaving a 2-inch border on one edge. Top with ¼ of the cucumber, ¼ of the romaine, and ¼ of the dressing. Fold one side of the tortilla up and over the fillings, fold in the edge with the border, and continue rolling the tortilla to the other side, making a tight bundle. Transfer the wrap to a plate or a platter, seam down. Repeat with the remaining tortillas.

Green Goddess Pasta

Serves 4

4 cloves garlic, minced

3 tablespoons refined coconut oil

6 tablespoons vegan butter

3 quarts water

About 5 teaspoons fine sea salt

8 ounces whole wheat or brown rice elbow macaroni

2 zucchini, halved lengthwise and cut into ¼-inch slices

1 broccoli crown, cut into bite-sized florets (about 2½ cups)

½ bunch (about 4 ounces) kale, cut into ½-inch strips

½ teaspoon pepper

¼ cup pine nuts

In a 1-quart saucepan over low heat, combine the garlic and coconut oil and cook, swirling occasionally, until the garlic is fragrant and starting to brown, about 3 minutes. Remove from the heat, add the butter, swirling until it melts, and set aside.

In a 4- to 6-quart stockpot over high heat, combine the water with about 1½ tablespoons salt. Bring the water to a boil, add the macaroni, and cook according to the package directions until about 1 minute shy of being done. Stir in the zucchini, broccoli, and kale. Cook until the vegetables are tender and the pasta is cooked, about 1 minute.

Drain the pasta mixture, reserving ½ cup of the pasta cooking water. Return the mixture to the pot and stir in the garlic butter, pepper, 3 tablespoons of the pine nuts, and the remaining ½ teaspoon of salt. Transfer the pasta to plates or a platter, garnish with remaining 1 tablespoon of pine nuts, and serve.

"Chicken" Square Meal with White Beans, Quinoa Pilaf, and Asparagus

Serves 6

1½ cups dried small white beans

2 cloves garlic, smashed

1 bay leaf

2 tablespoons extra virgin olive oil

1½ teaspoons fine sea salt

½ tablespoon refined coconut oil
   or safflower oil

1 cup quinoa

2 cups low-sodium vegetable stock

1 cup frozen mixed vegetables
   (no need to thaw)

6 vegan chicken cutlets

1 bunch (about 1 pound)
   asparagus, trimmed

1 lemon, cut into wedges,
   for garnish

In a 3-quart saucepan, combine the beans and enough cold water to cover by 1 inch. Cover and refrigerate for at least 8 hours or overnight. (Alternately, bring to a boil over high heat, cover, remove from heat, and let sit for 1 hour.) *

Drain the beans, return them to the saucepan, and cover with water by 1 inch. Add the garlic and bay leaf. Place the pot over high heat, bring to a boil, and reduce to a simmer. Cover and cook until the beans are tender, about 25 minutes. Remove from the heat, drain any water left in the pot, and stir in the olive oil and ¾ teaspoon of the salt.

Meanwhile, in a 2- to 3-quart saucepan over medium-high, melt the coconut oil. Add the quinoa and cook, stirring occasionally, until the quinoa is browned, about 5 minutes. Stir in the stock, the mixed vegetables, and ¼ teaspoon of the salt. Bring to a boil, reduce the heat to a simmer, cover, and cook until the stock is absorbed and the quinoa is tender, about 20 minutes.

While the beans and quinoa are cooking, cook the chicken according to package directions.

When everything is about 10 minutes from being done, in an 8- to 10-inch skillet over high heat, combine ½-inch of water and the remaining ½ teaspoon of salt and bring to a simmer. Add the asparagus and cook, turning occasionally and adjusting the heat to maintain a simmer, until crisp-tender, 3 to 5 minutes, depending on the size of the asparagus.

Transfer the chicken, beans, quinoa, and asparagus to 4 serving plates, dividing evenly. Garnish with lemon wedges and serve.

*For all you bitches in a rush: Instead of dried beans, you can use canned beans. Substitute 2 (15-ounce) cans of white beans. Place the beans and their liquid in 1- to 2-quart saucepan over medium heat. Bring to a simmer, reduce the heat to low, and cook until the beans are heated through, about 5 minutes. Cover and set aside until ready to serve— then, either drain the beans or serve them with a slotted spoon.

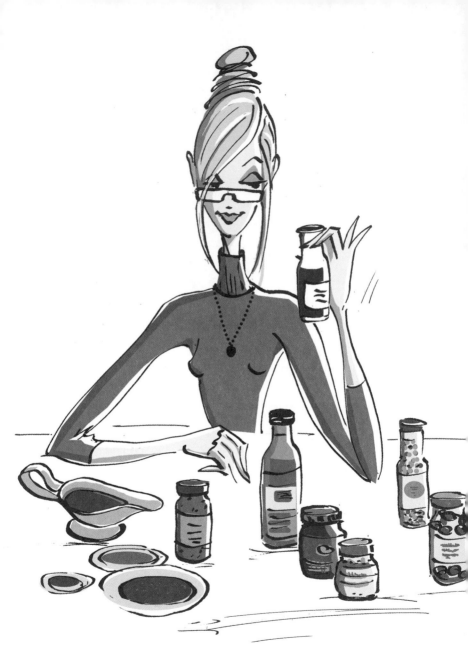

Divine Dressings,
SAUCES, AND
SUBSTITUTES

*If you have shitty taste buds from eating
poorly all these years, healthy food may not taste
so good to you. If that's the case, douse your
grub with any one of these gooey delights.*

Savory White Cream Sauce

Brown Gravy

Cheezy Sauce

Ranch Dressing

Thousand Island Dressing

Miso-Ginger Dressing

Agave-Dijon Spread

Agave-Dijon Dressing

Vegan Caesar Dressing

Basil Pesto

Sage Pesto

Basic Red Sauce

Super Simple Pizza Sauce

Tofu "Ricotta"

Marinated Tofu "Feta"

Savory White Cream Sauce

Makes about 2 cups

About 2 cups soy or rice milk

¼ cup refined coconut oil

½ onion, finely diced

¼ cup whole wheat pastry flour

½ teaspoon fine sea salt

¼ teaspoon white pepper

⅛ teaspoon ground nutmeg

In a 1-quart saucepan over low heat, heat 2 cups of soy milk until it's barely simmering (small bubbles will appear at the edges of the pan). Cover and set aside.

Heat the oil in a 2- to 3-quart saucepan over medium heat. Add the onion and cook, stirring occasionally, until tender, 4 to 6 minutes. Whisk in the flour and cook, whisking constantly, for 2 minutes. Slowly whisk in the hot milk and bring the mixture to a simmer. Reduce the heat to low and cook, whisking often, until the sauce is thick and no longer tastes of raw flour, 6 to 8 minutes. Remove from the heat and whisk in the salt, pepper, and nutmeg. If not using immediately, transfer the sauce to a bowl, cover with plastic wrap directly on the surface of the sauce, and use within 30 minutes. If the sauce gets too thick while it sits, whisk in a little more warm soy milk.

Brown Gravy

Makes about 2½ cups

¼ cup refined coconut oil

½ cup whole wheat pastry flour

2 to 2¼ cups low-sodium
vegetable stock

4 tablespoons Bragg's Liquid
Aminos (or 8 teaspoons tamari or
soy sauce)

Heat the oil in a 2- to 3-quart saucepan over medium heat. When the oil is almost completely melted, whisk in the flour. Cook, stirring often, until the mixture is browned and smells nutty, about 5 minutes. A little at a time, add 2 cups of the stock, whisking until smooth after each addition. Remove from the heat and whisk in the Bragg's Liquid Aminos (or tamari or soy sauce). Add more stock, if desired, until the gravy reaches the desired consistency. Serve hot, or cool, cover, and refrigerate for 3 or 4 days. Reheat gently, adding a little more stock or water if necessary.

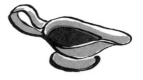

Cheezy Sauce

Makes about 2¾ cups

About 2 cups soy or rice milk

¼ cup refined coconut oil

¼ cup whole wheat pastry flour

8 ounces vegan cheese (cheddar, mozzarella, Jack, whatever you like, or a combination), shredded

½ teaspoon fine sea salt

¼ teaspoon white pepper

In a 1-quart saucepan over low heat, heat 2 cups of soy or rice milk until it's barely simmering (small bubbles will appear at the edges of the pan). Cover and set aside.

Heat the oil in a 2- to 3-quart saucepan over medium heat. Whisk in the flour and cook, whisking constantly, for 2 minutes. Slowly whisk in the hot milk and bring the mixture to a simmer. Reduce the heat to low and cook, whisking often, until the sauce is thick and no longer tastes of raw flour, 6 to 8 minutes. Remove from the heat and whisk in the cheese, salt, and pepper, stirring until the cheese melts (if necessary, return the pot to low heat). If not using immediately, transfer the sauce to a bowl, cover with plastic wrap directly on the surface of the sauce, and use within 30 minutes. If the sauce gets too thick while it sits, whisk in a little more warm soy or rice milk.

Ranch Dressing

Makes about 1¾ cups

1 cup vegan sour cream

½ cup soy milk

¼ cup safflower oil

1 tablespoon agave nectar

1 tablespoon granulated
  garlic powder

2 teaspoons chopped dill

1 teaspoon Dijon mustard

1 teaspoon fine sea salt

½ teaspoon onion powder

½ teaspoon cider vinegar

¼ teaspoon pepper

¼ teaspoon tamari or soy sauce

In a blender or a food processor, combine all ingredients and process until smooth. Set aside in the refrigerator overnight to allow the flavors to bloom. Store refrigerated for up to 1 week.

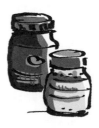

Thousand Island Dressing

Makes about 1⅓ cups

1 cup vegan mayonnaise

¼ cup ketchup

¼ cup sweet pickle relish

2 tablespoons tomato paste

3 tablespoons lemon juice

½ teaspoon fine sea salt

⅛ teaspoon cayenne

In a small bowl, whisk together all the ingredients. Use immediately, or cover and refrigerate for up to 1 week.

Eat. It. With. A. Spoon.

Miso Ginger Dressing

Makes about 1½ cups

¾ cup canola or safflower oil

¼ cup red miso

¼ cup water

2 tablespoons agave nectar

2 tablespoons rice wine vinegar

2 tablespoons grated fresh ginger

1 teaspoon sesame oil

In a small bowl, whisk together all the ingredients. Use immediately, or cover and refrigerate for up to 1 week.

This one's so good it can perk up even the lamest of salads.

Agave-Dijon Spread

Makes ½ cup

¼ cup agave nectar

¼ cup Dijon mustard

In a small bowl, whisk together the agave and mustard. Use immediately, or cover and refrigerate for up to 2 months.

> This spread can be used on all kinds of sandwiches, burgers, and "chicken."

Agave-Dijon Dressing

Makes about 1½ cups

¼ cup agave nectar

¼ cup Dijon mustard

⅔ cup extra virgin olive oil

¼ cup red wine vinegar or
   balsamic vinegar

2 cloves garlic, minced

½ teaspoon fine sea salt

½ teaspoon pepper

In a small bowl, whisk together all ingredients. Use immediately, or cover and refrigerate for up to 1 month.

> This would totally kick ass on a spinach salad.

Caesar Dressing

Makes 1½ cups

4 ounces silken tofu

6 tablespoons lemon juice

3 cloves garlic

2 tablespoons vegan
Parmesan cheese

½ tablespoon Dijon mustard

2 teaspoons vegan
Worcestershire sauce

½ teaspoon fine sea salt

½ teaspoon pepper

¼ teaspoon kelp powder (optional, to
give it an anchovy kind of flavor)

¾ cup extra virgin olive oil

In a food processor, combine the tofu, lemon juice, garlic, cheese, mustard, Worcestershire sauce, salt, pepper, and kelp powder, if using, and process until smooth. With the motor running, slowly drizzle in the olive oil. Use immediately, or cover and refrigerate for up to 1 week.

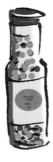

Basil Pesto

Makes about 1⅓ cups

¼ cup pine nuts

4 cloves garlic

3 cups fresh basil leaves

¼ cup vegan Parmesan cheese

½ teaspoon fine sea salt

⅛ teaspoon pepper

¾ cup extra virgin olive oil,
plus more for storing

In a food processor, combine the pine nuts and garlic and pulse to roughly chop. Add the basil and pulse to chop. Add the cheese, salt, and pepper and process into a paste. With the motor running, slowly pour in the olive oil, processing until the oil is fully combined. Use immediately or transfer to a small container, cover with a thin layer of olive oil, and store in the refrigerator for 3 to 4 weeks.

Sage Pesto

Makes about 1 cup

¼ cup whole almonds

2 cloves garlic

1½ cups fresh sage leaves

¾ cup fresh Italian parsley leaves

3 ounces (about ⅓ cup) soy
cream cheese

½ teaspoon fine sea salt

⅛ teaspoon pepper

⅔ cup extra virgin olive oil, plus
more for storing

In a food processor, combine the almonds and garlic and pulse to roughly chop. Add the sage and parsley and pulse to chop. Add the cream cheese, salt, and pepper and process into a paste. With the motor running, slowly pour in the olive oil, processing until the oil is fully combined. Use immediately or transfer to a small container, cover with a thin layer of olive oil, and store in the refrigerator for 3 to 4 weeks.

Basic Red Sauce

Makes about 7 cups

2 tablespoons refined coconut oil

1 onion, cut into ¼-inch dice

8 to 10 cloves garlic, minced

2 (28-ounce) cans crushed tomatoes

1 (6-ounce) can tomato paste

¼ cup fruity red wine (optional)

2 tablespoons finely

   chopped fresh basil

1 tablespoon finely

   chopped fresh oregano

½ teaspoon salt

⅛ teaspoon hot sauce, like

   Tabasco (optional)

1 tablespoon agave nectar

(optional)

Heat the coconut oil in a 4- to 6-quart stockpot over medium-low heat. Add the onion and cook, stirring occasionally, until tender, 6 to 8 minutes (adjust heat, if necessary, to avoid browning). Add the garlic and cook, stirring occasionally, 1 minute. Stir in the tomatoes and tomato paste, increase the heat to high, and bring to a boil. Remove from the heat and stir in the wine, if using, along with the basil, oregano, salt, and hot sauce (if using). Taste, and if the sauce is too acidic, stir in the agave. Use immediately or cover and refrigerate for up to 1 week or freeze for up to 2 months.

Super Simple Pizza Sauce

Makes about 1¾ cup

1 (14.5-ounce) can diced tomatoes

¼ cup tomato paste

2 cloves garlic

2 teaspoons red wine vinegar

1 teaspoon chopped fresh oregano

  or ½ teaspoon dried oregano

½ teaspoon fine sea salt

⅛ teaspoon pepper

⅛ teaspoon cayenne powder

In a food processor, combine all the ingredients and pulse to puree. Use immediately or cover and refrigerate for up to 1 week or freeze for up to 2 months.

Tofu "Ricotta"

Makes about 2 cups

14 to 16 ounces extra firm tofu,
  crumbled

3 cloves garlic

2 tablespoons extra virgin olive oil

1 tablespoon chopped fresh
  oregano or 1 teaspoon dried
  oregano

¾ teaspoon fine sea salt

In a food processor, combine the tofu, garlic, olive oil, oregano, and salt and pulse to puree. Use immediately or cover and refrigerate for up to 1 week.

> This is so similar to the real deal it makes us angry. Why is it so good? Why?

Marinated Tofu "Feta"

Makes about 3 cups

2 tablespoons extra virgin olive oil

1½ tablespoons lemon juice

1 teaspoon dried oregano

1 teaspoon fine sea salt

½ teaspoon crushed red pepper

14 to 16 ounces firm or extra firm
   tofu, cut into ½- or ¾-inch cubes

In a medium bowl, whisk together the olive oil, lemon juice, oregano, salt, and red pepper. Add the tofu and toss gently. Let marinate for at least 1 hour, stirring occasionally. Use immediately.

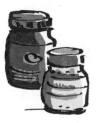

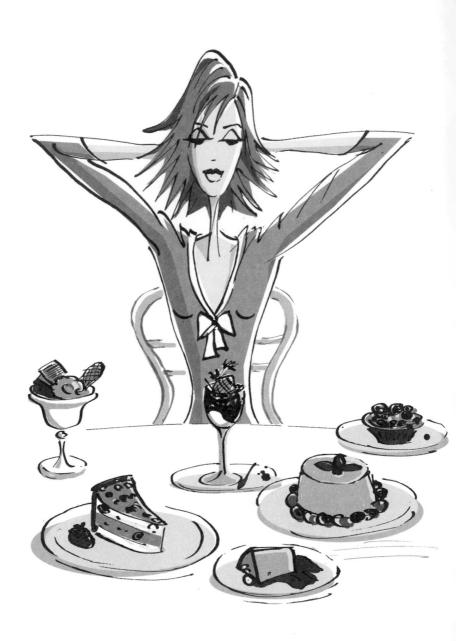

Happy
ENDINGS

If eating dessert is wrong, we don't want to be right.
Give us dessert, or give us death. Life without dessert is
like life without the sun. We never met a dessert we didn't
like. Clearly, we're totally fucking psychotic for dessert.

Chocolate Chip Cookies

Peanut Butter Potato Chip Cookies

Buttery Shortbread Cookies

Bitchtastic Brownies

Hot Fudge Brownie Sundaes

Cheezecake

Vanilla Cake with Frosting

Carrot Cake with Cream Cheese Frosting

Chocolate Suicide Cake

Dream Bars

Rice Pudding

Fresh Fruit Crisp

Chocolate Chip Cookies

Makes about 48

2½ cups whole wheat pastry flour

½ tablespoon baking soda

1 teaspoon fine sea salt

1½ cups evaporated cane sugar

1¼ cups refined coconut oil

¼ cup ice water

1 tablespoon molasses

½ tablespoon pure vanilla extract

1 (10- to 12-ounce) package vegan
  chocolate chips

1 cup chopped walnuts (optional)

Seriously. Can you stand these?

Preheat oven to 375°F. Line baking sheets with parchment.

In a medium bowl, sift together the flour, baking soda, and salt; set aside.

In the bowl of a stand mixer or in a large bowl with a hand mixer, combine the sugar and coconut oil, mixing on medium-high speed until creamy, about 3 minutes. Add the water, molasses, and vanilla, mixing until well combined. With the mixer on low speed, add the flour mixture in 3 to 4 additions, mixing each addition until almost fully incorporated. Add in the chocolate chips and the walnuts, if using, mixing until just combined.

Arrange 2-tablespoon-sized balls of cookie dough 2 inches apart on prepared baking sheets. Bake for 13 to 15 minutes, until the edges are slightly browned and the centers are set. Thoroughly cool on a cooling rack.

Peanut Butter Potato Chip Cookies

Makes about 40

2½ cups whole wheat pastry flour

2 teaspoons baking soda

¾ teaspoon fine sea salt

1½ cups evaporated cane sugar

1 cup refined coconut oil

1 cup all-natural peanut butter,
   chunky or smooth (whichever
   you prefer)

¼ cup ice water

1 tablespoon molasses

1 teaspoon pure vanilla extract

2 cups coarsely crushed potato chips

Preheat oven to 375°F. Line baking sheets with parchment.

In a medium bowl, sift together the flour, baking soda, and salt; set aside.

In the bowl of a stand mixer or in a large bowl with a hand mixer, combine the sugar, coconut oil, and peanut butter, mixing on medium-high speed until creamy, about 3 minutes. Add the water, molasses, and vanilla, mixing until well combined. With the mixer on low speed, add the flour mixture in 3 to 4 additions, mixing each addition until almost fully incorporated. Add the potato chips, mixing until just combined.

Arrange 2-tablespoon-sized balls of cookie dough 2 inches apart on prepared baking sheets. Press to about ¾-inch thick, then use the back of a fork to mark each cookie with a crosshatch pattern, if desired. Bake for 13 to 15 minutes, until the edges are slightly browned and the centers are set. Thoroughly cool on a cooling rack. Then eat enough to make yourself sick.

Buttery Shortbread Cookies

Makes about 36 cookies

1¾ cups whole wheat pastry flour

1 tablespoon coarse nutritional yeast

1 teaspoon fine sea salt

½ cup refined coconut oil, cut into
  pieces if in large chunks

½ cup powdered evaporated
  cane sugar

1 teaspoon pure vanilla extract

1 tablespoon orange juice

Preheat oven to 325 °F. Line baking sheets with parchment.

In a medium bowl, combine the flour, nutritional yeast, and salt; set aside.

In the bowl of a stand mixer or in a large bowl with a hand mixer, cream the coconut oil, mixing on medium-high speed for about 3 minutes. Add the sugar and beat until light and fluffy, about 2 minutes. Add the vanilla and orange juice, mixing until well combined. With the mixer on low speed, add the flour mixture in 3 to 4 additions, mixing until just combined. Transfer the dough to a work surface, shape it into a ¾-inch disk, cover with plastic wrap, and refrigerate until firm enough to roll out, 5 to 10 minutes.

Transfer the dough to a lightly floured work surface and roll out to ¼-inch thick. Cut into shapes and arrange on prepared baking sheets. Reroll the dough and cut into shapes one or two more times. Bake for 20 minutes, or until the edges are just starting to brown.

Bitchtastic Brownies

Makes 9 or 12

5 ounces unsweetened vegan
   chocolate, chopped

1¼ cups Sucanat
   (or other dry sweetener)

¾ cup silken tofu

6 tablespoons safflower oil, plus
   more for the pan

1 tablespoon pure vanilla extract

⅓ cup whole wheat pastry flour

2 tablespoons unsweetened
   cocoa powder

¼ teaspoon refined sea salt

Preheat oven to 350°F. Oil an 8 x 8 inch baking pan; set aside.

In the top of a double boiler or in a medium metal bowl set over a pot of gently simmering water, melt the chocolate, stirring just until smooth. Transfer the chocolate to a food processor and add the Sucanat, tofu, oil, and vanilla; process until smooth. Add the flour, cocoa powder, and salt, pulsing until just combined. Transfer the batter to the prepared pan, spreading it evenly. Bake for 30 minutes, until a toothpick inserted into the center comes out clean. Thoroughly cool on a cooling rack before cutting into 9 or 12 squares.

> Oh please, who are we kidding? Eat 'em while they're hot and burn your friggin' mouths off.

Hot Fudge Brownie Sundaes

Makes 4

4 ounces semi-sweet vegan
    chocolate, chopped

3 tablespoons vegan cream

4 Bitchtastic Brownies
    (preceding page)

1 pint vegan vanilla ice cream

2 tablespoons chopped toasted
    pecans

4 cherries with stems

In the top of a double boiler or in a medium metal bowl set over a pot of gently simmering water, melt the chocolate and cream, stirring just until smooth; set aside.

Arrange the brownies on plates. Top each with a scoop of ice cream then drizzle with the chocolate sauce (you may not need it all) and sprinkle with pecans, dividing evenly. Finish with a cherry on top, and serve.

Cheezecake

Serves 10 to 12

1½ cups vegan cookie crumbs
(see note on next page)

3 tablespoons refined coconut oil,
melted, or safflower oil

1 cup plus 7 tablespoons raw
(turbinado) evaporated cane
sugar (or other dry sweetener)

2 pounds tofu cream cheese

1 pound silken tofu

3 tablespoons arrowroot or
3 tablespoons plus 2 teaspoons
cornstarch

1 tablespoon pure vanilla extract

Zest and juice of 1 lemon

Fruit Glaze Topping
(optional, recipe follows)

Preheat oven to 325°F.

In a medium bowl, combine the cookie crumbs, oil, and 3 tablespoons of the sugar, stirring until the mixture is uniformly moist. Transfer to a 10-inch springform pan and press the mixture evenly into the bottom and 1 to 2 inches up the sides of the pan. Place the pan on a rimmed baking sheet and bake until the crust is lightly browned and dry, 15 to 20 minutes. Thoroughly cool on a cooling rack.

While the crust is cooling, increase the oven temperature to 350°F.

In the bowl of a food processor, combine about ¼ of the cream cheese and the tofu; process until smooth. Transfer the mixture to the bowl of a stand mixer or a large bowl with a hand mixer. Add the remaining cream cheese and the remaining 1¼ cups sugar and mix on medium speed until smooth.

In a small bowl, combine the arrowroot or cornstarch, vanilla, and lemon juice. Add this mixture, along with the lemon zest, to the cream cheese mixture, beating just until smooth. Pour the entire mixture into the cooled crust. Place the pan on the rimmed baking sheet and bake for 50 minutes.

When time is up, turn off the heat but leave the cheesecake in the oven until the edges are set and lightly browned but the center is still wobbly, about 60 minutes. Remove from the oven, run a knife around the edge of the crust, and let cool completely.

Cover and chill for at least 4 hours and up to a day before removing the sides of the pan. Just before serving, pour the glaze on top, if using, spreading it evenly.

To make cookie crumbs, start with whatever kind of vegan cookies you like—graham crackers, ginger snaps, chocolate wafers, whatever. Put a couple of handfuls in the food processor and pulse until they're finely ground. Repeat until you have 1½ cups (the number of cookies it takes depends on the size and density of the cookie).

FOR ALL YOU PSYCHO PERFECTIONISTS OUT THERE: There are a couple of tricks to reduce the chances of cracks on the top of a cheesecake. The most important is to not overcook it—trust that that wobbly center will indeed firm up after cooling and chilling. Another is to beat the filling only enough to make it smooth; overbeating increases the air in the filling which makes the cake rise, which can make the cake crack when it falls. A third trick is to run a knife around the edge of the cake right when it comes out of the oven. Still, even the best cooks will get a crack in their cheesecake now and then. So the best trick is to hide cracks with the fruit glaze.

FRUIT GLAZE TOPPING

1 cup all-fruit jam or preserves,
    whatever flavor you like
1 tablespoon arrowroot or
    3½ teaspoons cornstarch
    dissolved in ⅓ cup water

In a small saucepan over medium heat, whisk together the jam and the arrowroot mixture. Bring to a simmer, whisking until thickened and no longer milky-looking, about 3 minutes. Cool thoroughly before spreading on cooked, cooled, chilled cheesecake.

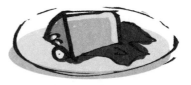

Vanilla Cake with Frosting

Serves 10 to 12

1 cup refined coconut oil,
    plus more for pans

4 cups whole wheat pastry flour,
    plus more for cake pans

1 tablespoon baking powder

½ teaspoon baking soda

¾ teaspoon fine sea salt

1⅓ cups rice or soy milk

1 cup silken tofu

⅓ cup safflower oil

1½ tablespoons vanilla extract

2 cups evaporated cane sugar
    (or other dry sweetener)

4 cups Vanilla or Chocolate Frosting
    (recipe follows)

Try not to eat the entire batch of frosting before you put it on the cake, pig.

Preheat oven to 350°F. Oil and flour two 9-inch cake pans and line the bottoms with parchment. Oil the parchment and dust the pans lightly with flour.

In a medium bowl, sift together the flour, baking powder, baking soda, and salt; set aside.

In a food processor, combine the milk, tofu, safflower oil, and vanilla; set aside.

In the bowl of a stand mixer or in a large bowl with a hand mixer, combine the coconut oil and sugar, mixing on medium-high speed until fluffy, 3 to 5 minutes. With the mixer on low speed, add the flour mixture in 3 additions, alternating with the tofu mixture, mixing until just combined.

Transfer the batter to the prepared pans and smooth the surfaces. Bake for 30 to 35 minutes, or until the cakes spring back when lightly touched in the center and begin to pull away from the sides of the pan. Cool on racks for 10 minutes. Unmold the cakes and return to racks to thoroughly cool.

Spread each cake with about ¼ of the Vanilla Frosting or Fudgy Chocolate Frosting. Stack the cakes, then use the remaining frosting to coat the sides of the cake and your boobs.

VANILLA FROSTING

Makes about 4 cups

½ cup refined coconut oil

8 to 10 tablespoons soy milk
   or nondairy creamer

2 teaspoons vanilla extract

¼ teaspoon salt

8 cups (about 2 pounds) powdered
   evaporated cane sugar

In the bowl of a stand mixer or in a large bowl with a hand mixer, cream the coconut oil, mixing on medium-high speed for about 3 minutes. Add 8 tablespoons of the milk or creamer, the vanilla, and salt, mixing until well combined. With the mixer on low speed, add the sugar, about ½ cup at a time. If the frosting seems too stiff, add 1 to 2 tablespoons more milk. Increase the speed to high and beat until smooth and fluffy, 1 to 2 minutes.

FUDGY CHOCOLATE FROSTING

Makes about 4 cups

14 tablespoons refined coconut oil

2 cups evaporated cane sugar

1½ cups unsweetened cocoa powder

1 cup soy creamer

½ teaspoon pure vanilla extract

¼ teaspoon fine sea salt

In a 2- to 3-quart saucepan over medium heat, melt the oil. Stir in sugar and cocoa powder. Gradually stir in creamer. Heat, stirring almost constantly, until mixture is smooth and hot, but not boiling. Remove from heat and stir in vanilla and salt. Set aside to cool to room temperature, until thick enough to spread.

Carrot Cake with Cream Cheese Frosting

Serves 10 to 12

1 cup safflower oil,
  plus more for the pans
3 cups whole wheat pastry flour,
  plus more for the pans
2 cups evaporated cane sugar
  (or other dry sweetener)
2 teaspoons baking powder
2 teaspoons baking soda
2 teaspoons cinnamon
1 teaspoon refined sea salt
2 cups finely shredded carrots
  (about 2 carrots)
2 cups unsweetened applesauce
2 teaspoons vanilla
1½ cups chopped walnuts
4 cups Vegan Cream Cheese
  Frosting (recipe follows)

Preheat oven to 350°F. Oil two 9-inch cake pans and line the bottoms with parchment. Oil the parchment and dust the pans lightly with flour.

In a large bowl, sift together the flour, sugar, baking powder, baking soda, cinnamon, and salt; set aside.

In another large bowl, combine the oil, carrots, applesauce, and vanilla, stirring until smooth. Stir in the flour mixture in 3 or 4 additions, mixing until barely combined. Add walnuts, stirring until just combined.

Transfer the batter to the prepared pans and smooth the surfaces. Bake for 35 to 40 minutes, or until the cakes spring back when lightly touched in the center and begin to pull away from the sides of the pan. Cool on racks for 10 minutes. Unmold the cakes and return to racks to cool thoroughly.

Spread each cake with about ¼ of the Vegan Cream Cheese Frosting. Stack the cakes, then use the remaining frosting to coat the sides of the cake.

VEGAN CREAM CHEESE FROSTING

Makes about 4 cups

12 ounces vegan cream cheese

1 tablespoon pure vanilla extract

¼ teaspoon salt

8 cups (about 2 pounds) powdered evaporated cane sugar (or other dry sweetener)

In the bowl of a stand mixer or in a large bowl with a hand mixer, combine the cream cheese, vanilla, and salt, mixing on medium speed until smooth. With the mixer on low speed, add the sugar, about ½ cup at a time. Increase the speed to high and beat until light and fluffy, 1 to 2 minutes.

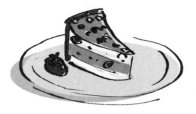

Chocolate Cake

Serves 12 to 16

¾ cup safflower oil, plus more
   for the pan

2 cups whole wheat pastry flour

1½ cups evaporated cane sugar

1 tablespoon cream of tartar

2 teaspoons baking soda

½ teaspoon fine sea salt

¾ cup vegan chocolate chips

1¼ cups soy milk

¾ cup unsweetened applesauce

½ tablespoon pure vanilla extract

4 ounces unsweetened vegan
   chocolate, chopped

1 tablespoon apple cider vinegar

2 cups Fudgy Chocolate Frosting
   (see page 171) (optional)

Write out your will while it's
cooking. It's just that good.

Preheat oven to 350°F. Oil a 13 x 9-inch baking pan; set aside.

In a large bowl, sift together the flour, sugar, cream of tartar, baking soda, and salt. Stir in the chocolate chips; set aside.

In a medium bowl, combine the oil, soy milk, applesauce, and vanilla, stirring until smooth; set aside.

In the top of a double boiler or in a medium metal bowl set over a pot of gently simmering water, melt the chocolate, stirring just until smooth.

Add the oil mixture into the flour mixture, stirring until smooth. Add the melted chocolate, stirring until smooth. Stir in the vinegar.

Transfer the batter to the prepared pan and smooth the surface. Bake for 40 to 45 minutes, until the cake springs back when lightly touched in the center and begins to pull away from the sides of the pan. Thoroughly cool on a cooling rack before frosting with Fudgy Chocolate Frosting.

Dream Bars

Makes 16 to 20

1½ cups vegan cookie crumbs
    (see note on page 168)

¼ cup refined coconut oil, melted

⅔ cups raw (turbinado) evaporated
    cane sugar, divided

⅔ cup peanut butter

2 tablespoons water

¼ cup vegan butter

¾ cup vegan chocolate chips

1 cup chopped walnuts

½ cup unsweetened shredded
    coconut

1 (13.5-ounce can) coconut milk

2 tablespoons agave nectar

1 tablespoon arrowroot or 3½
    teaspoons cornstarch dissolved
    into ½ tablespoon water

Preheat oven to 350° F.

In a medium bowl, combine the cookie crumbs, coconut oil, and ⅓ cup of the sugar, stirring until the mixture is uniformly moist. Transfer to a 13 x 9-inch baking pan and press the mixture evenly into the bottom.

Heat the peanut butter in a 1-quart saucepan over medium heat, stirring occasionally, until soft enough to pour. Drizzle the peanut butter over the cookie crumb mixture (don't worry about spreading it—just drizzle it evenly around).

In a 1-quart saucepan over medium heat, combine the remaining ⅓ cup of sugar and the water, stirring occasionally until the sugar is melted. Reduce the heat to low and continue to cook, swirling (not stirring) occasionally, until the mixture is a dark honey color. Remove the saucepan from the heat and swirl in the butter. Presto—you've got butterscotch sauce! Pour the butterscotch sauce evenly over the peanut butter. Top with chocolate chips, walnuts, and coconut, sprinkling each evenly.

In a small bowl, whisk together the coconut milk, agave, and arrowroot mixture. Pour the coconut milk mixture evenly over the toppings and bake for 30 minutes, until the coconut milk is set and the edges are browned. Thoroughly cool on a cooling rack before cutting into squares. For best results, set aside at room temperature overnight or in the refrigerator for 1 or 2 hours before serving.

Don't plan on sharing these with anyone. Hoard them for yourself.

Rice Pudding

Serves 4 to 6

2 cups soy creamer (or 1
    13.5-ounce can coconut
    milk plus ⅓ cup water)

1 cup water

1 cup medium-grain brown rice

Pinch fine sea salt

⅔ cup raisins, golden raisins,
    or a combination (optional)

2 tablespoons agave nectar

½ teaspoon pure vanilla extract

¼ teaspoon ground cinnamon

In a 2-quart saucepan over high heat, combine 1 cup of the creamer or coconut milk mixture, the water, rice, and salt. Bring to a boil, reduce the heat to a simmer, cover, and cook until the water is absorbed and the rice is almost tender, about 40 minutes.

Stir in the remaining 1 cup of creamer or coconut milk mixture, the raisins (if using), agave, vanilla, and cinnamon. Bring to a simmer and cook, stirring occasionally, until the raisins are plump and the rice is tender, about 5 minutes.

Spoon the pudding into bowls and let cool. Serve at room temperature or cover and refrigerate for about an hour before serving chilled.

If the pudding seems too thick, which can be the case if it's served cold, you can stir in a little soy milk or creamer.

Fresh Fruit Crisp

Serves 6

½ cup refined coconut oil,
  plus more for the pan

1 cup plus 2 tablespoons Sucanat,
  (or other dry sweetener)

½ cup plus 1 tablespoon whole
  wheat pastry flour

½ cup rolled oats

¾ teaspoon salt

1 teaspoon ground cinnamon

8 cups cored or pitted fresh fruit,
  one type or a combination,
  thinly sliced

2 tablespoons lemon juice

1 teaspoon pure vanilla extract

1 pint vegan vanilla ice cream
  (optional)

Preheat oven to 375°F. Oil an 8 x 8-inch baking pan.

In a medium bowl, combine 1 cup of the Sucanat, ½ cup of the flour, the oats, and ½ teaspoon of the salt. Using a pastry cutter or your fingertips, cut in the oil, mixing until the biggest pieces are the size of peas; set aside.

In a large bowl, combine the remaining 2 tablespoons of Sucanat, 1 tablespoon of flour, ¼ teaspoon of salt, and the cinnamon. Mix in the fruit, lemon juice, and vanilla.

Transfer the fruit to the prepared baking dish, spreading it evenly. Sprinkle on the topping. Bake for 30 minutes. If the fruit isn't yet tender (baking time will depend on the type of fruit), cover lightly with foil and bake for an additional 20 or 30 minutes.

Serve warm or at room temperature, topped with vegan vanilla ice cream, if using.

For the fresh fruit, use whatever is in season—whatever's the most ripe and full-flavored. Make it with apples in the fall, berries in the spring, and peaches in the summer. Apples will take the longer cooking time, pears a little less, and most other fruit will be done in 40 minutes—varying a little depending on ripeness and how thinly the fruit is sliced. Peeling isn't necessary.

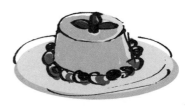

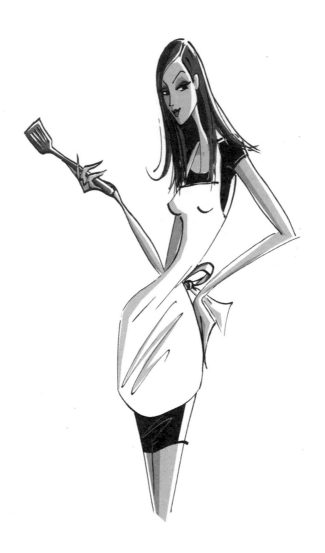

After-Dinner Mint

Food is the fuel that keeps us going. It supplies our bodies with energy and sustenance and literally makes life possible. But it's also so much more than that. It's the gateway to paradise. A gift from the heavens. Life's greatest pleasure. Every time we eat, we have the capacity to experience unparalleled ecstasy. Multiple times a day. So why do people forget to eat? Or eat standing up? Or grab something quick? Hell, it beats the shit out of us. We never do that stuff—we friggin' love eating more than anything else in the world. And we bask in the glory of every bite we take.

Eating is like a religious experience. And every meal is like an offering to your temple. So like you would for any place of worship, have reverence for your body. You shouldn't put garbage in your mouth any sooner than you'd go to church wearing crotchless panties. Now granted, sometimes you wear less than your Sunday best to church, and that's fine— God loves you, anyway. And sometimes you eat less than your best, and that's okay, too. But you wouldn't make a habit of dressing like crap for church and you shouldn't make a habit of eating crap, either.

We each get one body to last us an entire lifetime. And more than any other factor, food affects how well and for how long this body will serve us. So if you didn't care before, start caring now. Take the time to learn which foods are healthy and which aren't. And take the time to start enjoying everything you eat. Doing "it" standing up and "quickies" are for sex, not eating. So slow down, pick out a recipe, and sit down to a nice meal tonight. After dinner, you can have a quickie.

GLOSSARY

We know that for many of you, this is a whole new way of eating. So we salute your willingness to take it on—change is definitely hard. But it doesn't have to be scary. The more you know, the less intimidated you'll be. Knowledge is power.

Having said that, behold the glossary. (If there's an ingredient you're curious about that we don't define . . . look it up in a dictionary or online. Don't be a Needy Bitch.)

.....

Agave Nectar or Syrup: A sweetener, similar to honey, that comes from the Agave plant (where tequila happens to come from, too). It's less refined than regular sugar, so it doesn't contain processing chemicals. Buy the "raw" version.

Arrowroot: A starch flour made from the root of a plant. Like cornstarch, it's used as a thickener.

Bacon (vegan): Bacon alternative made from soy protein, wheat gluten, and other ingredients. Tastes like friggin' bacon, but doesn't encompass slaughtering a pig.

Bragg's Liquid Amino Acids: Tastes kinda like soy sauce, but contains no MSG. Made from soybeans and purified water. A must have with steamed-veggies and brown rice. Use Bragg's instead of soy sauce.

Cheese (vegan): A dairy-free cheese substitute that contains no milk, rennet (an enzyme from the stomach lining of calves), no casein (a milk protein), no whey (the liquid portion of milk that has curdled), and no other gross-out factor. Our favorite brand is Follow Your Heart.

Ener-G Egg Replacer: A vegan replacement for eggs in baking. Made from potato starch and tapioca flour to mimic eggs in recipes. Comes in powder form; just mix with water.

Evaporated Cane Sugar: Made from sugar cane, only the water has been removed. It's less processed than regular sugar, so it retains some nutrients.

Kelp Powder: Granules made from seaweed that lend a mild salty and/ or fishy flavor to dishes.

Mayonnaise (vegan): A dairy-, egg-, and cholesterol-free mayonnaise substitute. Our favorite brand: Follow Your Heart Vegenaise.

Nutritional Yeast Flakes: A non-leavening yeast that has a cheesy flavor. A food supplement that contains B vitamins and tastes great on salads, pizzas, and popcorn!

Oil (Coconut, Flaxseed, Hempseed): There is so much conflicting information regarding oils and there are so many different schools of thought. Here's the one we subscribe to: Oils are best when kept intact and not heated. So when you're using oil as a dressing or to add flavor to something after it's cooked, unrefined oil is best. If you can stand the taste, flaxseed oil is really good for you. Hempseed oil, cold-pressed extra virgin olive oil, and sesame seed oil are all good options, too. Heating oils, especially at high temperatures, can alter them into harmful toxic substances. However, a girl's gotta eat, and sometimes a girl's gotta heat her oil. With that said, some oils withstand heat better than others. Refined coconut oil is the best oil for high heat cooking. Canola oil and safflower oil are other decent options. (Never continue to use oil that has burnt or is smoking. And never save and re-use oil that you've already cooked with. Re-used fryer oil is just one of the reasons fast food is so damn bad for you.)

Parmesan (vegan): A Parmesan cheese substitute that is made without any dairy components. (Some companies make it with a soy-based version, and others make it with nutritional yeast and nuts.)

Pasta: Substitute regular, refined, white pasta with whole wheat, brown rice, or quinoa pasta. These are healthier alternatives that contain nutrients and fiber.

Rice Milk: Dairy-, lactose-, and cholesterol-free milk alternative made from brown rice, water, and a small amount of brown rice sweetener.

Seitan: High-protein meat substitute made from wheat gluten. The texture may freak you out at first, but keep trying it. Soon, you'll be hooked.

Soy Butter: A dairy-free butter substitute usually made from a blend of oils. Be sure to get the non-hydrogenated kind.

Soy Milk: Dairy-, lactose-, and cholesterol-free milk alternative made from soybeans. High in protein, vitamins, and minerals.

Sucanat: Sugar in its most natural form: SUgar CAne NATural. It's extracted from unrefined sugar cane where only the water has been removed. It retains the molasses, as well as the vitamins and minerals.

Tahini: Thick paste made from ground sesame seeds.

Tempeh: A vegan, meat-like alternative made from fermented soybeans. High in protein. The texture isn't really meaty—it's more nutty and grainy, kinda. Just shut up and try it.

Textured Soy Protein (also known as texturized vegetable protein): A meat substitute made from defatted soy flour that's compressed and processed into bite-size chunks. Generally, it needs to be rehydrated with water when using.

Tofu: Made from processed soybean curds. Good source of calcium and protein. Cholesterol-free, baby. Tofu is a total chameleon in recipes and can take on whatever flavor you want. It does take getting used to.

Turbinado: Made from 100 percent sugar cane. It's what's left after raw sugar has been washed, allowing the natural molasses to remain.

Vegan (noun): A person who abstains from eating cows, chickens, pigs, fish, eggs, and dairy. "I am a vegan."

Vegan (adjective): 1. The state of being with regard to not eating cows, chickens, pigs, fish, eggs, and dairy. "I am vegan." 2. A product free of animal ingredients. "Is that cookie vegan?"

Metric Conversion Tips

For all you bitches who use the metric system . . .

Generic Formulas for Metric Conversion

Ounces to grams	multiply ounces by 28.35
Pounds to grams	multiply pounds by 453.5
Cups to liters	multiply cups by .24
Fahrenheit to Centigrade	subtract 32 from Fahrenheit, multiply by five and divide by 9

Oven Temperatures

Degrees Fahrenheit	Degrees Centigrade	British Gas Marks
200°	93°	—
250°	120°	—
275°	140°	1
300°	150°	2
325°	165°	3
350°	175°	4
375°	190°	5
400°	200°	6
450°	230°	8

Metric Equivalents for Volume

U.S.	Imperial	Metric
⅛ tsp.	—	0.6 ml
½ tsp.	—	2.5 ml
¾ tsp.	—	4.0 ml
1 tsp.	—	5.0 ml
1½ tsp.	—	7.0 ml
2 tsp.	—	10.0 ml
3 tsp.	—	15.0 ml
4 tsp.	—	20.0 ml
1 Tbsp.	—	15.0 ml
1½ Tbsp.	—	22.0 ml
2 Tbsp. (⅛ cup)	1 fl. oz	30.0 ml
2½ Tbsp.	—	37.0 ml
3 Tbsp.	—	44.0 ml
⅛ cup	—	57.0 ml
4 Tbsp. (¼ cup)	2 fl. oz	59.0 ml
5 Tbsp.	—	74.0 ml
6 Tbsp.	—	89.0 ml
8 Tbsp. (½ cup)	4 fl. oz	120.0 ml
¾ cup	6 fl. oz	178.0 ml
1 cup	8 fl. oz	237.0 ml
(.24 liters)		
1½ cups	—	354.0 ml
1¾ cups	—	414.0 ml
2 cups (1 pint)	16 fl. oz	473.0 ml
4 cups (1 quart)	32 fl. oz	(.95 liters)
5 cups	—	(1.183 liters)
16 cups (1 gallon)	128 fl. oz	(3.8 liters)

Metric Equivalents for Weight

U.S.	Metric
1 oz	28 g
2 oz	58 g
3 oz	85 g
4 oz (¼ lb.)	113 g
5 oz	142 g
6 oz	170 g
7 oz	199 g
8 oz (½ lb.)	227 g
10 oz	284 g
12 oz (¾ lb.)	340 g
14 oz	397 g
16 oz (1 lb.)	454 g

Metric Equivalents for Butter

U.S.	Metric
2 tsp.	10.0 g
1 Tbsp.	15.0 g
1½ Tbsp.	22.5 g
2 Tbsp. (1 oz)	55.0 g
3 Tbsp.	70.0 g
¼ lb. (1 stick)	110.0 g
½ lb. (2 sticks)	220.0 g

Metric Equivalents for Length

(USE ALSO FOR PAN SIZES)

(USE ALSO FOR PAN SIZES)

U.S.	Metric
¼ inch	.65 cm
½ inch	1.25 cm
1 inch	2.50 cm
2 inches	5.00 cm
3 inches	6.00 cm
4 inches	8.00 cm
5 inches	11.00 cm
6 inches	15.00 cm
7 inches	18.00 cm
8 inches	20.00 cm
9 inches	23.00 cm
12 inches	30.50 cm
15 inches	38.00 cm

INDEX